The Lost Book of Herbal Remedies

400 Essential Herbal Remedies for Everyday Wellness

Brett Axford

© 2024 Brett Axford. All rights reserved.

Please note that unauthorized reproduction, storage, retrieval, transmission, or distribution of this publication is strictly prohibited without the publisher's prior written consent, as outlined in the 1976 US Copyright Act, Sections 107 and 108.

Limitation of Liability/Disclaimer of Warranty:

The publisher and the author provide no guarantees regarding the accuracy or completeness of the contents of this work. They specifically disclaim all warranties, including those related to fitness for a specific purpose. There are no warranties that can be created or extended through sales or promotional materials. Please note that the advice and strategies provided may not be suitable for all situations. This work is sold with the understanding that the publisher is not providing medical, legal, or other professional advice or services. If you need professional assistance, it is advisable to seek the services of a competent professional person. The publisher and author are not responsible for any damages that may occur. Please note that the inclusion of an individual, organization, or website as a citation or potential source of further information in this work does not imply endorsement by the author or publisher. The information or recommendations provided by these sources are not necessarily endorsed. Additionally, it is important for readers to note that any websites mentioned in this work may have undergone changes or become unavailable since the time of writing.

ISBN: 978-1-326-74501-1

Author: Brett Axford

Book Title: The Lost Book of Herbal Remedies: 400 Essential Herbal Remedies for Everyday Wellness

TABLE OF CONTENTS

INTRODUCTION	1
How to Harvest Herbs	2
How to Dry Herbs	2
Encapsulating Powdered Herbs	3
Herbal Water Infusions: Cold and Hot Methods	4
Teas	5
Decoctions	5
Steps for Making a Decoction:	5
Oil Infusions	6
Tinctures/Extracts	7
HERBAL REMEDIES	11
Digestive Health Herbs	11
Immune System Support Herbs	14
Skin Health Herbs	17
Nervous System & Mental Health Herbs	20
Respiratory Health Herbs	23
Liver and Detoxification Herbs	26
Cardiovascular Health Herbs	29
Hormonal Health Herbs	32
Blood Sugar & Weight Management Herbs	35
Anti-inflammatory & Pain Relief Herbs	38
Antioxidant & Anti-Aging Herbs	41
Anti-Viral & Antibacterial Herbs	44
Bone and Joint Health Herbs	47
Kidney and Urinary Health Herbs	50
Stress and Anxiety Relief Herbs	53
Hair and Scalp Health Herbs	56
Circulatory Health Herbs	59
Mood & Cognitive Support Herbs	62
Sexual Health & Libido Herbs	65
Eye Health Herbs	68
Antiseptic & Healing Herbs	71
Antidepressant & Mood-Boosting Herbs	73
Menstrual Health & Women's Reproductive Health Herbs	76
Anti-Cancer & Tumor-Fighting Herbs	79
Detox & Cleansing Herbs	83
Heart Health & Circulatory System Herbs	86
Fertility and Sexual Health Herbs	89
Antifungal & Antimicrobial Herbs	92
Liver Support & Detox Herbs	96
Respiratory Support & Cough Remedies	99

DIGESTION & GUT HEALTH HERBS	102
IMMUNITY-BOOSTING & IMMUNE SUPPORT HERBS	104
BRAIN & COGNITIVE FUNCTION HERBS	107
NERVOUS SYSTEM & RELAXATION HERBS	110
ANTI-OBESITY & WEIGHT LOSS HERBS	113
DETOXIFICATION & LIVER SUPPORT HERBS	116
BLOOD SUGAR REGULATION & INSULIN SUPPORT HERBS	119
RESPIRATORY SUPPORT & COUGH RELIEF HERBS	122
SKIN HEALTH & ANTI-AGING HERBS	124
HAIR GROWTH & SCALP HEALTH HERBS	127

INTRODUCTION

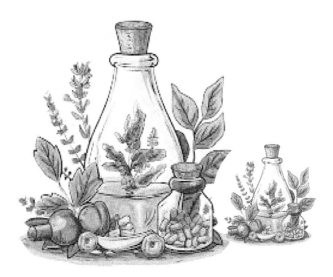

Modern medicine, when compared to the vast timeline of human history, is relatively recent. While the pharmaceutical industry is a modern development, the use of medicine has spanned thousands of years. Early medicines were derived from natural sources, harnessing the healing properties of what nature offers.

Herbal remedies, which have been used throughout history, continue to be effective today. Despite a decline in widespread knowledge about these natural treatments, they remain as valuable as ever. This book aims to help readers rediscover and share this ancient wisdom.

Although the pharmaceutical industry often dismisses herbal medicine, it is, in fact, the precursor to much of contemporary medicine. Many modern drugs attempt to replicate the properties of natural substances. Most so-called "medicines" are synthetic versions of compounds found in nature. This chemical modification is often necessary, as patent laws prevent the patenting of naturally occurring substances. As a result, pharmaceutical companies create synthetic alternatives, many of which come with significant side effects.

However, this does not mean modern medicine and herbal treatments cannot coexist. They can, and often do. In many cases, herbs can serve as more affordable and lower-risk alternatives to prescription drugs, benefiting both our health and finances.

In a post-apocalyptic scenario, herbal remedies may be our primary form of medicine. If modern manufacturing and distribution systems break down, we will have to rely on locally grown plants. Many individuals who possess knowledge of herbal medicine are already cultivating these plants and preparing them for medicinal use.

An added benefit of growing and using your own herbs, rather than purchasing supplements from a store, is that you control the freshness and growing conditions of the plants. The sooner you harvest and prepare your herbs, the more potent they tend to be. Additionally, by making your own herbal mixtures, you can be certain of the contents—free from additives or fillers—ensuring that you only use the herbs you need.

How to Harvest Herbs

Herbal medicines originate from living plants, which may not always align with the traditional image of "herbs." They can come from trees, flowers, roots, mushrooms, lichens, and more. While many people cultivate herb gardens, others gather medicinal plants from the wild. Developing the skill to identify medicinal plants in nature is highly valuable.

When identifying plants, it is essential to refer to images that show the plants at various stages of their life cycle. A reliable plant identification guide specific to your area is crucial for accuracy.

Many people are familiar with flower identification, but without flowers, identifying plants becomes challenging. Since most plants only flower briefly, the window for harvesting is limited.

Before harvesting herbs, it's important to understand how the plant will be used and which part of the plant holds medicinal properties. Don't assume that the entire plant contains the same active compounds; often, only the leaves or flowers are useful, while in other cases, the bark or roots may be required.

It's best to harvest herbs early in the day, after the dew has evaporated but before the sun's heat can diminish the essential oils. Whenever possible, avoid harvesting the entire plant unless it is necessary to do so.

For leaves, cut small branches to make drying easier. For flowers, wait until they are fully open and harvest them as soon as possible after blooming. If you're collecting seeds, allow them to mature fully and the seed pods to dry on the stem before harvesting. This book provides specific harvesting instructions for most herbs.

When cutting stems, such as when harvesting stinging nettle, ensure that at least a few inches of the stem, with two sets of leaves, are left intact to allow the plant to regenerate. With many plants, such as basil, you can safely cut up to a third of the plant without damaging it. Always aim to reseed, replant, and care for the wild environment. Harvest with respect and mindfulness.

How to Dry Herbs

Traditionally, herbs are dried by air without using additional heat. To dry them, bundle the stems together with string or a rubber band and hang them in a warm, dry location. The most common method is to hang the bundles upside down by the stems.

For those drying large quantities of herbs or doing so regularly, drying racks can be useful. However, you can achieve the same result by hanging the herbs from a coat hanger, a nail in the wall, or a curtain rod over a window. Alternatively, you can spread flowers or leaves on a cookie sheet or pizza pan and let them dry.

When collecting seeds, tie a paper bag over the bundled stems and hang them. The bag will catch the seeds as the seed pods dry and release them.

This drying method can take up to three weeks, though it often occurs more quickly, depending on the plant and its moisture content. For herbs that dry slowly, like rosemary, it's easier to strip the leaves from the stems and spread them on a drying rack. The leaves' natural coating retains moisture, so ensuring they are fully dried before storing is essential.

If you have a dehydrator with temperature control, you can also use it to dry herbs. Ideally, the dehydrator should have a fan to circulate warm air, ensuring even drying. To prevent overheating or burning the herbs, use the lowest possible temperature. I have successfully used this method several times. When using a dehydrator, monitor the herbs closely to avoid over-drying.

Once the herbs are fully dried, remove the leaves from the stems. For smaller leaves, lightly pinch the stem between your thumb and forefinger and slide your hand down the stem to strip the leaves off. For larger leaves with thicker stems, cut or pinch them off individually, as close to the leaf as possible.

Store your dried herbs in sealed glass jars until ready for use.

Encapsulating Powdered Herbs

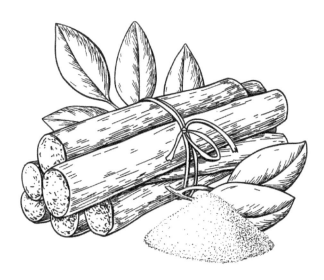

When you visit a health food store to purchase herbs, you'll often find them available in powdered form and encapsulated for convenience. This method is especially useful when administering herbs to individuals who are not familiar with herbal remedies.

There are two primary ways to encapsulate herbs, but the first step is to convert them into powder. You can easily achieve this by grinding the herbs in a food processor or an electric coffee grinder. For a more traditional approach or if you are without electricity, you can use a mortar and pestle.

If you plan to create herbal mixtures, you will need a scale to accurately measure the herbs. Be sure to mix the powdered herbs thoroughly to ensure that each capsule contains a consistent amount of the desired herbal concentration.

Herbal capsules come in three sizes: "0," "00," and "000." You can fill them either by hand or with a simple filling machine. The most cost-effective method is to fill them by hand. Begin by placing the powder in a large bowl. Open the capsules one at a time, then scoop the powder into both halves of the capsule, aiming to fill them reasonably full. Afterward, press the capsule halves together, allowing the powder to compress as the capsule closes. Although this method is effective, it can be tedious and time-consuming, so you may want to enlist some help or have company while performing the task.

Capsule Filling Machines

To streamline the process, you can invest in a simple capsule-filling machine. These machines are available in sizes for 50 or 100 capsules and must be selected to match the size of the capsules you're using. The machine consists of several plates with holes to hold the capsule halves and a base.

Start by separating the capsules, placing each half into separate bowls. The longer, thinner half goes into the base plate of the machine. Use a funnel-like device to pour the capsule halves onto the plate, then gently shake the machine until the halves fall into the holes, positioning them for filling. Repeat the same process with the top plate.

Once the capsule halves are in place, pour a quantity of powdered herbs onto the base plate. Use the provided scraper to move the powder around, ensuring it fills the capsules. Afterward, scrape off any excess powder. To close the capsules, position the top plate over the bottom plate. The machine includes aligning pins to ensure proper alignment of the halves. Then, press down on the plates several times to secure the capsules. Finally, remove the filled capsules and store them in a jar.

Herbal Water Infusions: Cold and Hot Methods

Both tea and coffee are types of infusions, typically made with hot water. While cold versions of these beverages are often initially infused with hot water and then chilled in the refrigerator or with ice, it is also possible to make cold-infused coffee and tea, though the process is slower. Cold infusion requires more time to extract the flavors and properties of the herbs or beans into the water.

The infusion process simply extracts the active compounds from the plant material, whether leaves or beans, into the water. This method can be applied to almost any herb.

The most common way to infuse herbs is by making a hot tea. Herbal teas can be prepared using single herbs, but it is more typical to create blends of herbs that complement each other to address specific health concerns.

Hot infusions have the advantage of extracting more of the essential compounds from plant tissues because the heat helps break down the cell walls, resulting in a stronger infusion. However, hot infusions can also release undesirable compounds, such as those that contribute to a bitter taste. In such cases, a cold infusion may be a better option. Mucilaginous herbs, such as lemon balm, marshmallow, slippery elm, and comfrey, tend to extract more effectively when infused cold, as the mucilage remains intact.

Sun tea is one of the most popular types of cold infusion. To make it, you can either leave the herbs loose (to strain later) or place crushed leaves in a cheesecloth or muslin bag, which can be tied to the top of your jar or cup. For tea, most people use 1 to 2 teaspoons of dried herbs for every 8 ounces (250ml) of water. If using dried herbs, it is helpful to moisten them before placing them in the cold infusion, though this step is not necessary with fresh herbs. Allow the infusion to sit for at least 48 hours to fully extract the beneficial compounds.

Teas

Herbal tea is one of the most popular methods for using herbs for medicinal purposes. As mentioned earlier, herbal tea is a "hot infusion," which is highly effective at extracting the beneficial compounds from many herbs. Unlike cold infusions, which require more time, hot infusions can be prepared in just a few minutes.

Teas can be made from either fresh or dried herbs, and each form will produce slightly different results. Since each herb reacts differently depending on whether it is fresh or dried, it's important to understand the best approach for each individual herb or herbal blend.

Decoctions

A decoction is a concentrated form of a hot infusion or tea, making it highly effective for herbs that release their beneficial compounds slowly, such as woody parts or roots. It is also an excellent method for creating a more concentrated herbal supplement, especially for individuals like children, animals, or those who may not consume enough of a hot infusion to receive its full benefits.

To prepare a decoction, begin with cold distilled or purified water. The use of cold water is essential to ensure the maximum extraction of beneficial nutrients from the herbs. It's best to prepare the decoction in an earthenware, glass, or glazed ceramic pot to avoid the interaction between metal pots and the astringent herbs, which can alter the flavor.

Use a ratio of 1 ounce (28g) of dried herbs to 16 ounces (500ml) of water. Decoctions are typically made in small quantities, as they should be consumed within a couple of days, since they don't store well in the refrigerator for more than three days. If you need to store a decoction longer, keep it in a tightly sealed container or freeze it (ice cube trays work well). You can also add two tablespoons of alcohol (such as vodka, rum, or brandy) per 8 ounces of decoction to enhance preservation.

Steps for Making a Decoction:

1. Crush, chop, or grind the herbs into small pieces and place them in the cold water in your cooking pot.
2. Allow the herbs to soak in the cold water for a few hours.
3. Cover the pot and bring it to a slow boil. Once boiling, reduce the heat to a simmer.
4. Continue simmering until the liquid volume is reduced by half (approximately 15-20 minutes).
5. Strain the mixture using cheesecloth. After it cools, squeeze the herbs to extract any remaining liquid.
6. Transfer the decoction into a jar with a lid for storage. Use it within 48 hours or freeze it.

Decoctions are four times more concentrated than teas. Adults in good health can typically consume up to 1 cup of decoction three times a day, depending on the herb. Children's dosages should be adjusted based on their weight.

Double Decoctions:

Double decoctions follow the same process as regular decoctions but are simmered longer until the liquid is reduced to a quarter of its original volume, which increases the medicinal concentration. For most herbs, adults should take no more than 1 tablespoon of a double decoction, while children should have up to ½ teaspoon. Double decoctions are particularly useful for extracting compounds from shredded bark and dried roots, which release their beneficial compounds more slowly. When working with these herbs, allow them to soak in cold water for 12 hours before bringing them to a boil and simmering.

Oil Infusions

The methods outlined below for hot and cold infusions are used to extract herbs into oil. In cold extractions, "cold" refers to room temperature, and this method relies on time to infuse the herbs. It typically takes 6 to 8 weeks to infuse herbs into a carrier oil at room temperature. In contrast, the "hot" method involves gently warming the oil to speed up the extraction process, which is necessary for certain herbs. However, it is important to avoid overheating the oil, as excessive heat can alter the chemical composition of the herbs' active properties.

Carrier Oils and Infusion Methods:

For cold oil infusions, start with dried herbs (with a few exceptions), as moisture can cause the oil to spoil or mold. Many carrier oils can be used, but I prefer organic olive oil due to its stability at various temperatures, cost-effectiveness, and suitability for salve-making. Always purchase organic oils from reputable sources with strict labeling standards, such as those in California. Other good carrier oils include sweet almond oil, coconut oil (though its consistency changes with temperature), jojoba oil, baobab oil, tamanu oil, castor oil, grapeseed oil, argan oil, avocado oil, apricot kernel oil, emu oil, and others. Rendered fats, like bear fat, can also be used.

Cold Oil Infusion:

1. Tear or crush the dried herbs and lightly pack them into a clean, sterilized glass jar. Fill the jar about one-third full with the dried herbs (for certain herbs, like cottonwood buds, you may fill it more than half-full).

2. Pour your high-quality organic olive oil (or another plant-based oil) over the herbs, filling the jar to within ½ inch (1.25 cm) of the top. Mix well to remove any air bubbles. Cap the jar and label it with the herb name and date.

3. Store the jar for 6 to 8 weeks. Avoid storing it for longer than 8 to 10 weeks, as the oil may go rancid (cottonwood buds are an exception). To speed up the infusion process for some herbs, you can gently heat the jar in a water bath on low for a day or two, then store it for the remaining 6 to 8 weeks.

4. After 6 to 8 weeks, strain the herbs using cheesecloth or a tincture press. Squeeze the cheesecloth to extract all the herbal oil. Transfer the oil into a clean, sterile container. This infused oil can be used directly for medicinal purposes or to make salves. It typically lasts 1 to 2 years.

Hot Oil Infusion:

For hot oil infusion, use a crockpot with a "warm" or very low setting, or a stovetop water bath on low heat. This method works well for infusing multiple oils at once.

1. Place dried herbs into your jar (for herbs like cottonwood buds or Usnea, fill the jar more than halfway).
2. Pour high-quality organic olive oil (or another natural oil) over the herbs, filling the jar to within ½ inch (1.25 cm) of the top. Stir well to remove air bubbles. Cap the jar and label it with the herb name and date.
3. Place the jars in the crockpot and cook on low for 4 to 7 days, depending on the herb, ensuring that the water level in the crockpot or water bath remains consistent. For fresh herbs, leave the jar caps off to allow moisture to evaporate and prevent water from entering the jars.
4. Once the infusion has cooled, strain the herbs using cheesecloth or a tincture press. Transfer the oil into a clean, sterile container. This infused oil can be used directly for medicinal purposes or to make salves. It typically lasts 1 to 2 years.

Tinctures/Extracts

Tinctures are concentrated herbal extracts made by infusing herbs in a base of alcohol, vinegar, or glycerin. Alcohol is the most commonly used solvent because it effectively extracts essential oils and most of the other chemical compounds that water can also draw out. (Some herbs may require a dual extraction process—first in water, then in alcohol—to fully access all their medicinal properties.)

However, the primary advantage of alcohol-based tinctures is their rapid absorption into the body. The alcohol allows the tincture to pass through the stomach wall and even absorb through the mouth, sending the herbal compounds directly into the bloodstream rather than undergoing digestion.

Another significant benefit of tinctures is their long shelf life. When stored in an airtight container, tinctures remain potent indefinitely. The alcohol prevents microbial growth, making decomposition unlikely, though evaporation of the alcohol is the main concern.

To create a tincture, you will need a consumable alcohol that is at least 80 proof (40% alcohol). Vodka is the preferred choice due to its neutral flavor, but rum, gin, brandy, or whiskey can also be used. Alternatively, apple cider vinegar or food-grade vegetable glycerin can work, though these options are often less effective and have a shorter shelf life.

Instructions for Making a Tincture:

1. Fill a glass jar 1/3 to 1/2 full with dried herbs, ensuring the herbs are not packed tightly. The quantity of herbs depends on their surface area and how easily they release their active compounds. If using fresh herbs, use double the amount compared to dried.

2. Pour the alcohol over the herbs, leaving about ½ inch (1.25 cm) of headspace. Stir well to combine.

3. Seal the jar with a lid, label it with the herb name and date, and store it in a cool, dry place. The tincture should extract for 4 weeks to 6 months, with 2 months being ideal for most herbs. Shake the jar daily if possible.

4. After the extraction period, strain out the herbs and transfer the finished tincture into a clean container. Tinctures are highly shelf-stable due to the alcohol and can last up to 7 years. Many people transfer tinctures to dropper bottles for ease of use, but any small glass bottle will suffice. The typical adult dose is ½ to 1 teaspoon, while children should take about ¼ to 1/3 of the adult dose, based on their weight.

Double Extractions

A double extraction combines both a tincture and a decoction, commonly used for mushrooms and lichens. Recent research has highlighted the medicinal properties of various mushrooms. For instance, using only a water-based decoction for Reishi Mushroom extracts polysaccharides (including beta-glucans) and glycoproteins, but it does not extract triterpenes (such as ganoderic acid in Reishi), as these compounds are not water-soluble. To fully extract all medicinal compounds, both water and alcohol are necessary.

The double extraction process requires both alcohol and water. There are two methods to choose from, depending on the herbalist's preference. Both methods result in a tincture with an alcohol content of 25% to 30% or higher. If your final product appears cloudy, it is simply due to the polysaccharides coming out of solution, and shaking before use will resolve this.

Method #1: Starting with the Alcohol Extraction

You can scale down this recipe as needed. You'll need:

- 8 ounces (224g) of dried mushrooms or lichen
- 24 ounces (750ml) of 80–100 proof alcohol (40-50% alcohol)
- 16 ounces (500ml) of distilled water

Instructions:

1. Place the diced dried mushrooms into a quart-sized (1-liter) canning jar, filling it halfway. Add alcohol to within ½ inch (1.25 cm) of the top. Stir, seal the jar, and shake it daily for two months. After this period, strain out the alcohol and set it aside.

2. Prepare the decoction: Add 16 ounces (500ml) of water and the mushrooms to a ceramic or glass pot with a lid. Simmer the mixture until half the water evaporates, leaving about 8 ounces (250ml) of decoction. This may take a few hours. Add more water if necessary to maintain the simmer.

3. Let the decoction cool and strain out the mushrooms. Combine the decoction with the alcohol tincture (you should have about 24 ounces or 710ml of tincture) to complete the double extraction. The final product, with an alcohol content of 30%, should be shelf-stable for many years when stored in a sealed container.

Method #2: Starting with the Water Extraction

For this method, a small crockpot works well, but you can also place the herbs and water in a jar and immerse it in a water bath (either in a crockpot on low or on the stove). The recipe can also be scaled down. You'll need:

- 8 ounces (230g) or more of dried mushrooms or lichen
- 24 ounces (710ml) of 80–100 proof alcohol
- 16 ounces (500ml) of distilled water

Instructions:

1. Cut the herbs into small pieces and place them into the crockpot with the distilled water. Stir well, then cover and cook on the lowest setting for 3 days, reducing the liquid to about 8 ounces (250ml) of medicinal decoction.
2. Once cooled, transfer the herb-water mixture to a large glass jar. Add the alcohol while the mixture is still warm, but not hot. Ensure the jar is large enough to hold 24 ounces (710ml) of alcohol, or split the mixture between two jars.
3. Seal the jar tightly, label and date it, and allow it to macerate for 6 to 8 weeks. Shake the jar daily.
4. After the extraction period, strain the herbs using cheesecloth or carefully decant the tincture. Store the final tincture in a tightly sealed jar, labeled and dated.

Distillation

Distillation is a process used to extract essential oils from herbs and other plants. While not all plants yield essential oils, distillation is one of the most reliable methods for extracting them from those that do.

However, distillation is best suited for individuals who plan to produce large quantities of essential oils, as it requires a significant investment in equipment and a large amount of plant material. Since the yield of essential oil from plants is relatively small, a larger still is necessary to make the effort worthwhile. For most people, purchasing organic essential oils from a trusted supplier may be a more practical option.

There are three primary types of distillation, each requiring slight variations in the still:

- **Water Distillation:** The herbs are submerged in water, which is then boiled. This method works best for herbs that do not break down easily.
- **Water and Steam Distillation:** This method differs from water distillation in that a rack is placed inside the still to hold the herbs above the water, allowing steam to contact the plant material. This technique extracts essential oils more quickly than water distillation.
- **Direct Steam Distillation:** This requires a specialized still where steam is generated in a separate chamber and then injected into the main chamber, where the herbs are placed below a rack. This

allows for lower temperatures, reducing the risk of heat damage to the essential oil. This method is commonly used in commercial production, especially for oils like rosemary and lavender.

Distillation requires significant expertise, as the amounts of plant material, distillation times, and temperatures must be carefully tailored to both the still and the specific herb being processed.

HERBAL REMEDIES

Digestive Health Herbs

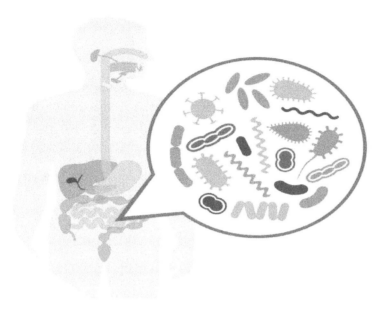

A healthy digestive system is essential for overall well-being. The digestive process is responsible for breaking down food, absorbing nutrients, and eliminating waste. When digestion becomes sluggish or imbalanced, it can lead to discomfort, bloating, indigestion, and other gastrointestinal issues. Fortunately, nature offers a variety of herbs that have been used for centuries to support digestive health. These herbs help to soothe, stimulate, and balance the digestive process, promoting a more efficient and comfortable gut.

Peppermint (*Mentha piperita*)

Peppermint is one of the most widely recognized and effective herbs for digestive health. Known for its cooling and soothing properties, peppermint relaxes the muscles of the digestive tract, helping to relieve indigestion, bloating, and gas. Its active compound, menthol, has a calming effect on the stomach and intestines, making it an excellent choice for easing symptoms of irritable bowel syndrome (IBS) and nausea.

- **How to Use**: Peppermint tea is a popular choice, made by steeping 1–2 teaspoons of dried leaves in hot water for 5–10 minutes. Peppermint oil capsules can also be used to target digestive discomfort more directly, with 1–2 capsules taken after meals.
- **Dosage**: 1–2 cups of tea per day or 1–2 peppermint oil capsules (enteric-coated) as directed.

Ginger (*Zingiber officinale*)

Ginger is a powerful herb known for its ability to improve digestion, alleviate nausea, and reduce inflammation. It stimulates the production of digestive enzymes and bile, helping to break down food more efficiently. Ginger also aids in relieving bloating and discomfort caused by indigestion and gas. Its anti-inflammatory properties make it especially beneficial for individuals with inflammatory bowel conditions.

- **How to Use:** Fresh ginger can be added to teas, smoothies, or meals. For digestive support, 1–2 teaspoons of freshly grated ginger can be steeped in hot water to make a soothing tea. Ginger supplements are also available in capsule form for convenience.
- **Dosage:** 1–2 teaspoons of fresh ginger or 1–2 capsules (500 mg) per day.

Fennel (*Foeniculum vulgare*)

Fennel is an herb known for its ability to relieve bloating, gas, and indigestion. It works by promoting the smooth movement of food through the digestive tract and helping to relax the muscles of the stomach and intestines. Fennel also stimulates the production of bile, which helps with fat digestion, making it a useful herb for those with sluggish digestion.

- **How to Use:** Fennel seeds can be chewed after meals to help with digestion or steeped into a tea by adding 1–2 teaspoons of seeds to hot water. Fennel essential oil can also be diluted and massaged onto the abdomen to relieve bloating and cramps.
- **Dosage:** 1–2 cups of fennel tea per day or 1–2 teaspoons of fennel seeds after meals.

Chamomile (*Matricaria chamomilla*)

Chamomile is a gentle, soothing herb often used to calm the digestive system and promote relaxation. It is particularly effective for relieving nausea, indigestion, and mild stomach cramps. Chamomile's anti-inflammatory properties help to reduce irritation in the digestive tract, making it ideal for those suffering from conditions like gastritis or IBS.

- **How to Use:** Chamomile is most commonly consumed as a tea, with 1–2 teaspoons of dried chamomile flowers steeped in hot water for 5–10 minutes. It is best consumed before or after meals to calm the stomach and promote digestion.
- **Dosage:** 1–2 cups of chamomile tea per day, particularly before bed for its calming effects.

Slippery Elm (*Ulmus rubra*)

Slippery elm is a demulcent herb, which means it forms a protective layer over the mucous membranes of the digestive tract. This soothing effect helps to alleviate symptoms of heartburn, acid reflux, and ulcers. Slippery elm is also known to support the healing of the gastrointestinal lining, making it useful for individuals with chronic digestive issues.

- **How to Use:** Slippery elm is commonly available as a powder, which can be mixed with water or added to smoothies. A common dosage is to mix 1 tablespoon of slippery elm powder in a glass of warm water to create a soothing drink.
- **Dosage:** 1–2 tablespoons of slippery elm powder per day, typically in the morning or before meals.

Dandelion Root (*Taraxacum officinale*)

Dandelion root is a powerful digestive herb that acts as a mild diuretic, promoting the elimination of waste and excess fluid. It also supports liver function, which plays a key role in digestion by filtering toxins and producing bile. Dandelion root stimulates appetite, supports healthy digestion, and can help alleviate constipation by encouraging regular bowel movements.

- **How to Use**: Dandelion root is commonly consumed as a tea or tincture. To make dandelion root tea, steep 1–2 teaspoons of dried root in hot water for 5–10 minutes. Dandelion root supplements are also available in capsule form.
- **Dosage**: 1–2 cups of dandelion root tea per day or 1–2 capsules of dandelion root (500 mg) as directed.

Marshmallow Root (*Althaea officinalis*)

Marshmallow root is another demulcent herb that soothes and protects the mucous membranes of the digestive tract. It is particularly effective for relieving irritation caused by acid reflux, gastritis, and ulcers. The mucilage in marshmallow root helps to reduce inflammation and promote healing of the gastrointestinal lining.

- **How to Use**: Marshmallow root is most commonly used in tea form, with 1–2 teaspoons of dried root steeped in hot water. It can also be taken as a tincture or capsule.
- **Dosage**: 1–2 cups of marshmallow root tea per day or 1–2 capsules (500 mg) as directed.

Licorice Root (*Glycyrrhiza glabra*)

Licorice root is known for its ability to soothe and protect the digestive system. It helps to relieve indigestion, heartburn, and gastric ulcers by promoting the secretion of mucus, which helps to protect the stomach lining. Licorice also has anti-inflammatory properties, making it beneficial for individuals with inflammatory digestive disorders.

- **How to Use**: Licorice root can be consumed as a tea, made by steeping 1–2 teaspoons of dried root in hot water for 5–10 minutes. It can also be taken in capsule or tincture form.
- **Dosage**: 1–2 cups of licorice root tea per day or 1–2 capsules (500 mg) per day. Note: Licorice should be used with caution in individuals with high blood pressure.

Artichoke (*Cynara scolymus*)

Artichoke is a highly effective herb for promoting healthy digestion, particularly for those struggling with bile production and fat digestion. It stimulates the liver to produce bile, which helps break down fats and improves overall digestion. Artichoke is also known to support healthy cholesterol levels and liver function.

- **How to Use**: Artichoke extract is available in capsule or liquid form, and artichoke tea can be made from the leaves. Artichoke can also be eaten in its whole form, such as in salads or steamed as a vegetable.
- **Dosage**: 1–2 capsules of artichoke extract (500 mg) or 1–2 cups of artichoke tea per day.

Immune System Support Herbs

A strong, resilient immune system is vital for defending the body against infections, illnesses, and diseases. While a balanced diet, regular exercise, and adequate sleep are essential for immune health, certain herbs can provide powerful support to enhance the body's natural defense mechanisms. For centuries, traditional herbal medicine has utilized the healing properties of plants to boost immunity and prevent illness. These herbs can help activate immune cells, reduce inflammation, and provide antimicrobial protection, ensuring your body remains equipped to fight off pathogens effectively.

Echinacea (*Echinacea purpurea*)

Echinacea is one of the most widely used herbs for immune support. This powerful plant contains compounds that stimulate the activity of white blood cells, which play a critical role in fighting infections. Echinacea has been shown to reduce the duration and severity of common colds and respiratory infections by enhancing the body's natural immune response. It also has antiviral and anti-inflammatory properties, making it effective in preventing and treating viral infections.

- **How to Use:** Echinacea is commonly consumed as a tea, tincture, or in capsule form. The dried flowers or root can be steeped in hot water to make a tea, or you can take standardized capsules for a concentrated dose.
- **Dosage:** For tea, use 1–2 teaspoons of dried Echinacea flowers or root per cup of water, steeped for 5–10 minutes. For tinctures, 20–30 drops can be taken 2–3 times per day. Echinacea capsules typically range from 300–500 mg, taken 2–3 times a day during cold or flu season.

Elderberry (*Sambucus nigra*)

Elderberry is known for its potent antiviral properties and has been used traditionally to treat cold and flu symptoms. The berries of this shrub contain anthocyanins and flavonoids, which help boost immune function and reduce the severity of viral infections. Studies have shown that elderberry extract can help reduce the duration of flu symptoms and speed up recovery. It also acts as an anti-inflammatory, helping to ease the symptoms of colds, coughs, and respiratory infections.

- **How to Use:** Elderberry can be consumed as a syrup, tincture, or in capsules. It is also available as a dried berry that can be steeped to make tea.
- **Dosage:** For elderberry syrup, 1–2 tablespoons daily can help prevent illness. During illness, take 1 tablespoon every 2–3 hours. Capsules typically contain 500 mg of elderberry extract, taken 1–2 times per day.

Astragalus (*Astragalus membranaceus*)

Astragalus is an adaptogenic herb known for its ability to enhance immune function and improve the body's ability to resist stress. It helps strengthen the immune system by stimulating the production of white blood cells and enhancing the body's overall defense mechanisms. Astragalus is often used to support the body during times of immune weakness, such as during recovery from illness or when experiencing chronic stress. It also has anti-inflammatory and antioxidant properties, supporting long-term immune health.

- **How to Use**: Astragalus is commonly taken as a tea, tincture, or capsule. The root can be boiled to make a soothing tea, or tinctures can be taken for a more concentrated dose.
- **Dosage**: For tea, steep 1–2 teaspoons of dried root in hot water for 5–10 minutes. For tincture, take 20–30 drops 2–3 times daily. Astragalus capsules generally contain 500–1000 mg, taken 1–2 times per day.

Andrographis (*Andrographis paniculata*)

Andrographis is a powerful herb traditionally used in Ayurvedic and Traditional Chinese Medicine for its immune-boosting and anti-inflammatory effects. It is particularly known for its ability to reduce the severity of cold and flu symptoms, such as fever and sore throat. Andrographis helps enhance the body's immune response by stimulating the production of cytokines, which are proteins that help regulate immune function. Studies have shown that it can also reduce the duration of upper respiratory infections.

- **How to Use**: Andrographis is typically available in capsule, tablet, or tincture form. The capsules provide a convenient, concentrated dose of this herb.
- **Dosage**: Standard dosages for Andrographis range from 400–1200 mg daily, taken in divided doses. For tinctures, 20–30 drops can be taken 2–3 times a day.

Garlic (*Allium sativum*)

Garlic has been celebrated for its medicinal properties for thousands of years, particularly for its role in supporting the immune system. Garlic contains allicin, a sulfur compound that has powerful antimicrobial and antiviral properties. It helps activate immune cells, promotes healthy circulation, and supports the body's ability to fight infections. Garlic also has anti-inflammatory and antioxidant effects, further enhancing immune function.

- **How to Use**: Fresh garlic can be consumed raw, chopped, or crushed to release its beneficial compounds. Garlic supplements are also widely available in capsule or tablet form.
- **Dosage**: To reap the full immune benefits, consume 1–2 cloves of raw garlic daily. If using supplements, a typical dosage is 300–1000 mg of garlic extract, taken 1–2 times per day.

Ginger (*Zingiber officinale*)

Ginger is a well-known herb for its ability to soothe digestive discomfort, but it also plays a significant role in boosting immune health. Ginger has potent anti-inflammatory and antioxidant properties, which help strengthen the immune system and fight infections. Its ability to promote circulation and reduce inflammation makes it particularly helpful for colds, flu, and respiratory infections. Ginger also enhances the production of white blood cells, improving the body's ability to defend against pathogens.

- **How to Use**: Fresh ginger can be added to teas, smoothies, or meals. Ginger supplements in capsule or tincture form are also effective.

- **Dosage:** Fresh ginger tea can be made by steeping 1–2 teaspoons of grated ginger in hot water for 5–10 minutes. Ginger supplements typically contain 500–1000 mg, taken 1–2 times per day.

Reishi Mushroom (*Ganoderma lucidum*)

Reishi mushrooms are revered in Traditional Chinese Medicine for their ability to enhance overall immune health. They are considered immune modulators, meaning they help regulate and balance the immune system. Reishi supports the production of immune cells and enhances the body's response to infections and inflammation. It is particularly useful for boosting immunity during periods of chronic stress or illness, making it an excellent choice for long-term immune support.

- **How to Use:** Reishi mushrooms can be consumed in the form of powders, capsules, or tinctures. Reishi mushroom extract is commonly used for concentrated doses.
- **Dosage:** For powder, 1–2 teaspoons per day is typically recommended, either added to warm beverages or smoothies. Reishi mushroom capsules typically range from 500–1000 mg per dose, taken 1–2 times daily.

Turmeric (*Curcuma longa*)

Turmeric is a renowned anti-inflammatory herb, primarily known for its active compound curcumin. Curcumin has been shown to enhance immune function by modulating the activity of immune cells, reducing inflammation, and supporting the body's defense mechanisms. It also has potent antioxidant effects, helping to protect cells from oxidative stress and damage. Turmeric supports both innate and adaptive immunity, making it a versatile herb for overall immune health.

- **How to Use:** Turmeric can be taken in various forms, including fresh root, powdered form, or as a supplement. A popular method of consumption is through turmeric tea or golden milk, made by adding turmeric powder to warm milk (or a dairy-free alternative).
- **Dosage:** For powdered turmeric, 1–2 teaspoons daily is a typical dosage. Curcumin supplements range from 500–1000 mg, taken 1–2 times daily.

Olive Leaf (*Olea europaea*)

Olive leaf extract is a powerful herb known for its antimicrobial, antiviral, and immune-boosting properties. It contains oleuropein, a compound that helps stimulate the immune system and fight infections. Olive leaf extract has been shown to be particularly effective against viral infections, including the flu, colds, and respiratory infections. It also helps reduce inflammation and supports cardiovascular health.

- **How to Use:** Olive leaf extract is commonly available in capsules, tablets, or tincture form. It can also be consumed as a tea.
- **Dosage:** Olive leaf capsules typically contain 500 mg of extract, taken 1–2 times per day. For tinctures, 20–30 drops can be taken 2–3 times daily.

Skin Health Herbs

Healthy, radiant skin is often a reflection of overall well-being, but many factors—such as environmental pollution, stress, poor diet, and aging—can take a toll on the skin. While skincare products may offer temporary relief, herbs provide long-lasting, natural solutions to nourish and protect the skin from within. Many herbs are rich in antioxidants, vitamins, and anti-inflammatory compounds that promote healthy skin, soothe irritation, and fight acne, eczema, and other common skin conditions. By incorporating these herbs into your daily routine, you can support your skin's natural ability to heal and regenerate.

Aloe Vera (*Aloe barbadensis miller*)

Aloe vera is one of the most beloved herbs for skin care, renowned for its soothing, cooling, and healing properties. This succulent plant is rich in vitamins, minerals, and antioxidants that help to nourish the skin and support its healing process. Aloe vera gel is often used topically to relieve sunburn, minor cuts, burns, and skin irritation. It also has moisturizing properties, making it ideal for dry or sensitive skin.

- **How to Use:** Aloe vera gel can be extracted directly from the plant and applied to the skin. Aloe vera juice is also available and can be consumed to promote skin hydration and improve skin health from within.
- **Dosage:** Apply aloe vera gel to the skin as needed, especially after sun exposure or skin irritation. For internal use, 1–2 ounces of aloe vera juice per day can help promote skin hydration and support overall health.

Calendula (*Calendula officinalis*)

Calendula, also known as marigold, is a powerful herb for promoting skin healing and reducing inflammation. Calendula has antimicrobial and anti-inflammatory properties, making it ideal for treating skin conditions like acne, eczema, cuts, bruises, and rashes. It also helps to stimulate collagen production, which can improve skin elasticity and promote a youthful appearance. Calendula is often used in creams, ointments, and oils for topical application.

- **How to Use:** Calendula can be used topically in creams, oils, or tinctures. For skin irritation or wounds, apply calendula oil or ointment directly to the affected area.
- **Dosage:** Use calendula oil or cream as needed for skin conditions. When using as a tincture, take 10–15 drops diluted in water 2–3 times per day for internal support.

Chamomile (*Matricaria chamomilla*)

Chamomile is widely known for its calming properties, not just for the mind but for the skin as well. Its anti-inflammatory and antioxidant properties make chamomile an excellent herb for soothing irritated, inflamed, or sensitive skin. Chamomile helps calm conditions like eczema, rosacea, and acne, and it promotes healing for minor skin wounds. Its gentle nature makes it suitable for all skin types, including sensitive and inflamed skin.

- **How to Use:** Chamomile can be used as a tea for internal benefits, or its essential oil can be diluted with a carrier oil and applied to the skin. Chamomile tea bags can also be used as a compress to reduce skin inflammation and puffiness.

- **Dosage:** Drink 1–2 cups of chamomile tea daily to promote skin healing from within. For topical use, mix 2–3 drops of chamomile essential oil with a carrier oil like jojoba or coconut oil and apply to the skin.

Lavender (*Lavandula angustifolia*)

Lavender is another versatile herb with multiple benefits for skin health. Its antiseptic, anti-inflammatory, and calming properties make it ideal for treating a variety of skin issues, from acne to minor burns and insect bites. Lavender oil can also help balance oil production in the skin, which can be beneficial for both dry and oily skin types. It's relaxing properties can help alleviate stress, which is often a contributing factor to skin flare-ups such as acne or eczema.

- **How to Use:** Lavender essential oil can be diluted with a carrier oil and applied to the skin to reduce inflammation and promote healing. Lavender tea can also be consumed to reduce stress and improve skin health indirectly.
- **Dosage:** For topical use, mix 2–3 drops of lavender oil with a carrier oil and apply to the affected area. You can also drink 1–2 cups of lavender tea for its calming benefits.

Gotu Kola (*Centella asiatica*)

Gotu kola is a powerful herb used in traditional medicine for wound healing and skin regeneration. Rich in triterpenoids, gotu kola enhances collagen production and improves skin elasticity, making it a popular choice for reducing the appearance of scars, stretch marks, and fine lines. Gotu kola is also known to support the healing of burns, cuts, and other skin damage, promoting faster recovery and healthier skin.

- **How to Use:** Gotu kola is typically consumed in the form of capsules, powders, or extracts. It can also be applied topically in creams or ointments to accelerate the healing process.
- **Dosage:** Take 500–1000 mg of gotu kola extract 1–2 times per day. For topical use, apply gotu kola cream or ointment to scars or wounds as directed.

Turmeric (*Curcuma longa*)

Turmeric, particularly its active compound curcumin, has been recognized for its potent anti-inflammatory, antioxidant, and antimicrobial properties. Curcumin helps to calm skin inflammation, reduce acne breakouts, and improve skin tone. It also supports the healing of wounds and scars and is often used to brighten the complexion. Turmeric is especially effective for conditions like psoriasis, eczema, and acne due to its ability to reduce redness and irritation.

- **How to Use:** Turmeric can be taken internally as a tea or supplement, or applied topically in face masks or creams. A turmeric face mask made with honey and yogurt can help reduce acne inflammation and brighten the skin.
- **Dosage:** For internal use, consume 1–2 teaspoons of turmeric powder daily, either in a warm drink or as part of your meals. For topical use, mix turmeric powder with honey or yogurt and apply as a mask 1–2 times per week.

Witch Hazel (*Hamamelis virginiana*)

Witch hazel is an astringent herb that has long been used for its ability to tone and tighten the skin. It is effective at reducing swelling, inflammation, and redness, making it an ideal remedy for acne, eczema, and other skin irritations. Witch hazel also has mild antiseptic properties, which help to cleanse the skin and prevent bacterial infections. It is often used as a natural remedy for acne treatment.

- **How to Use:** Witch hazel is most commonly used as a topical astringent or toner. It can be applied directly to the skin with a cotton ball or used in creams and lotions.
- **Dosage:** Apply witch hazel extract or toner to the skin 1–2 times daily, particularly on acne-prone areas.

Rosehip (*Rosa canina*)

Rosehip is a potent herb packed with vitamin C, antioxidants, and essential fatty acids, all of which support healthy skin and promote collagen production. Rosehip oil is commonly used in skincare products for its ability to reduce the appearance of scars, wrinkles, and stretch marks. Its hydrating properties make it ideal for dry or mature skin, and it helps improve overall skin texture and tone.

- **How to Use:** Rosehip oil is often used as a facial serum or moisturizer. It can be massaged into the skin directly or mixed with other oils like jojoba or argan oil for added hydration.
- **Dosage:** Apply a few drops of rosehip oil directly to the skin after cleansing, ideally in the evening. Rosehip tea can also be consumed for additional internal benefits, with 1–2 cups per day.

Burdock Root (*Arctium lappa*)

Burdock root is a detoxifying herb that helps purify the blood and promote clear skin. Its anti-inflammatory and antibacterial properties make it particularly effective for conditions like acne, eczema, and psoriasis. Burdock root helps to cleanse the skin by removing toxins from the bloodstream, which can reduce inflammation and promote a healthier complexion. It is also used to treat skin infections and irritation.

- **How to Use:** Burdock root can be consumed as a tea, tincture, or supplement. It is also available in topical preparations for direct application to the skin.
- **Dosage:** Drink 1–2 cups of burdock root tea per day or take 500–1000 mg of burdock root in capsule form 1–2 times per day.

Nervous System & Mental Health Herbs

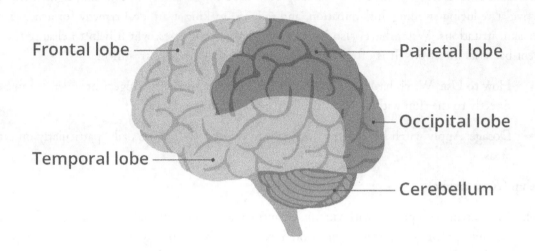

In today's fast-paced world, maintaining a balanced nervous system and optimal mental health can be a challenge. Stress, anxiety, depression, insomnia, and cognitive decline are common issues that many individuals face. Fortunately, nature offers a wealth of powerful herbs that can help restore harmony to the nervous system, calm the mind, and improve overall mental health. These herbs are rich in compounds that support neurotransmitter function, regulate stress hormones, and promote relaxation, mood stability, and cognitive clarity.

Using herbs to support the nervous system is a holistic approach to mental well-being. These herbs can be taken in various forms, such as teas, tinctures, capsules, or even incorporated into your daily diet. Below are some of the most effective herbs for supporting mental health and nervous system function.

Ashwagandha (*Withania somnifera*)

Ashwagandha is an adaptogenic herb renowned for its ability to help the body manage stress. It has been used in Ayurvedic medicine for thousands of years to promote balance and vitality. Ashwagandha works by reducing cortisol levels (the stress hormone) and supporting the adrenal glands, making it an excellent remedy for anxiety, stress, and fatigue. It also improves sleep quality and has been shown to enhance cognitive function and memory.

- **How to Use**: Ashwagandha is available in powder, capsule, and tincture form. The powder can be mixed into smoothies or warm milk for a calming bedtime drink, while capsules and tinctures offer a more convenient method of consumption.
- **Dosage**: A typical dosage is 300–500 mg of standardized extract, taken once or twice a day. For powder, 1 teaspoon per day is recommended, often taken with warm water or milk before bedtime.

Valerian Root (*Valeriana officinalis*)

Valerian root is one of the most well-known herbs for promoting relaxation and improving sleep quality. Its calming effects make it an effective remedy for insomnia, anxiety, and nervous tension. Valerian works by increasing the levels of gamma-aminobutyric acid (GABA), a neurotransmitter that helps reduce brain activity and induce relaxation. It is commonly used to calm the nervous system and support restful sleep.

- **How to Use**: Valerian root can be taken in capsule, tablet, or tincture form. It is also available as a tea, although it has a strong, earthy taste.
- **Dosage**: For sleep, 400–900 mg of valerian root extract is typically taken 30 minutes to an hour before bedtime. For tinctures, 20–30 drops in water or tea can be taken before sleep.

St. John's Wort (*Hypericum perforatum*)

St. John's Wort is widely recognized for its mood-boosting properties, particularly in the treatment of mild to moderate depression. The active compounds in this herb, including hypericin and hyperforin, help regulate serotonin levels in the brain, which can improve mood, reduce feelings of sadness, and alleviate symptoms of depression. It also has mild anxiolytic (anxiety-reducing) effects and can help stabilize emotional well-being.

- **How to Use**: St. John's Wort is available in capsule, tablet, or tincture form. It is important to note that this herb can interact with certain medications, so it is essential to consult with a healthcare provider before using it.
- **Dosage**: The standard dosage for St. John's Wort extract is 300 mg, taken 1–3 times daily. For tinctures, 20–30 drops 2–3 times a day are commonly used.

Lemon Balm (*Melissa officinalis*)

Lemon balm is a calming herb known for its ability to reduce anxiety and promote relaxation. It has a mild sedative effect that can help with nervous tension, stress, and insomnia. Lemon balm is often used to improve mood, reduce anxiety-induced restlessness, and support overall emotional well-being. It also has cognitive-enhancing properties, improving memory and mental clarity.

- **How to Use**: Lemon balm can be consumed as a tea, tincture, or in capsule form. The tea is particularly soothing before bed to help induce relaxation.
- **Dosage**: For tea, use 1–2 teaspoons of dried lemon balm leaves per cup of water, steeped for 5–10 minutes. For tinctures, take 20–30 drops up to 3 times per day. Capsules typically contain 300–500 mg, taken 1–2 times daily.

Rhodiola (*Rhodiola rosea*)

Rhodiola is another adaptogen that helps the body adapt to stress and enhance mental performance. Known as "the Arctic root," rhodiola has been shown to reduce fatigue, improve cognitive function, and alleviate symptoms of anxiety and depression. It works by balancing the levels of serotonin, dopamine, and norepinephrine, which are essential for mood regulation and cognitive clarity. Rhodiola is particularly effective for those dealing with mental fatigue or burnout.

- **How to Use**: Rhodiola is commonly taken in capsule or tincture form. The capsule form is convenient and provides a consistent dosage.
- **Dosage**: The recommended dose of Rhodiola extract is 200–400 mg daily. For tinctures, 30–40 drops can be taken once or twice a day.

Ginkgo Biloba (*Ginkgo biloba*)

Ginkgo biloba is primarily known for its benefits to cognitive function and memory. It works by improving blood circulation to the brain, which enhances mental clarity, focus, and memory retention. Ginkgo also has neuroprotective properties, which can help reduce the risk of cognitive decline and support mental agility in older adults. It is also known to help manage symptoms of anxiety by reducing oxidative stress in the brain.

- **How to Use:** Ginkgo biloba is available in capsules, tablets, and liquid extract forms. It is often used as a memory booster and cognitive enhancer.
- **Dosage:** A typical dosage is 120–240 mg of standardized ginkgo extract daily, divided into two or three doses.

Passionflower (*Passiflora incarnata*)

Passionflower is a mild sedative herb that helps calm anxiety and promote restful sleep. It is particularly effective for individuals experiencing nervous tension, insomnia, or stress-related symptoms. Passionflower works by increasing GABA levels in the brain, which calms the nervous system and helps to induce relaxation. It is often used in combination with other herbs, such as valerian or chamomile, for enhanced sedative effects.

- **How to Use:** Passionflower can be consumed as a tea, tincture, or in capsules. The tea is gentle and soothing, especially before bed.
- **Dosage:** For tea, use 1–2 teaspoons of dried passionflower leaves per cup of water. Steep for 5–10 minutes. For tinctures, 20–30 drops can be taken before bed to promote sleep.

Holy Basil (Tulsi) (*Ocimum sanctum*)

Holy Basil, also known as Tulsi, is a revered herb in Ayurvedic medicine for its ability to reduce stress, promote mental clarity, and support overall emotional balance. It is an adaptogen that helps the body adapt to physical, emotional, and mental stress, improving resilience and mood. Holy basil has also been shown to reduce symptoms of anxiety, depression, and cognitive fatigue, while supporting immune health and promoting mental clarity.

- **How to Use:** Holy basil is commonly available as a tea, tincture, or in capsules. It is often consumed as a daily tonic to promote overall well-being.
- **Dosage:** For tea, 1–2 teaspoons of dried holy basil leaves per cup of hot water. For capsules, a typical dosage is 500 mg of holy basil extract, taken once or twice a day.

Skullcap (*Scutellaria lateriflora*)

Skullcap is a calming herb traditionally used to ease anxiety, reduce nervous tension, and improve sleep quality. It has mild sedative properties that can help reduce stress and promote a sense of tranquility. Skullcap works by calming the nervous system and enhancing the effects of other calming herbs, such as valerian or passionflower.

- **How to Use:** Skullcap is commonly used as a tea, tincture, or in capsule form. It is especially beneficial when used in combination with other calming herbs.

- **Dosage**: For tea, steep 1–2 teaspoons of dried skullcap in hot water for 5–10 minutes. For tinctures, take 20–30 drops 2–3 times daily.

Respiratory Health Herbs

The health of our respiratory system is crucial for overall well-being, as it provides the oxygen our bodies need to function optimally. However, factors such as pollution, allergies, colds, respiratory infections, and chronic conditions like asthma or bronchitis can hinder proper breathing and lung function. Fortunately, nature offers a variety of herbs that can support respiratory health, soothe irritated airways, and promote clear, easy breathing. Whether you are seeking relief from congestion, enhancing lung function, or simply maintaining respiratory wellness, there are herbs that can help.

Respiratory health herbs are rich in compounds that help reduce inflammation, loosen mucus, fight infection, and support lung repair. These herbs can be consumed in various forms, including teas, tinctures, capsules, and inhalants, allowing for flexible and effective use. Below are some of the most effective herbs for respiratory health.

Eucalyptus (*Eucalyptus globulus*)

Eucalyptus is one of the most widely used herbs for respiratory health, particularly for relieving congestion and promoting easier breathing. Its active compound, eucalyptol (also known as 1,8-cineole), has anti-inflammatory, antimicrobial, and decongestant properties. Eucalyptus works by opening the airways, reducing inflammation, and thinning mucus, making it an excellent remedy for conditions like colds, bronchitis, asthma, and sinus infections.

- **How to Use**: Eucalyptus oil can be inhaled directly or used in steam inhalation to clear nasal passages and improve airflow. It is also commonly used in chest rubs and balms to relieve congestion.
- **Dosage**: For steam inhalation, add 2–3 drops of eucalyptus essential oil to a bowl of hot water and inhale the steam for 5–10 minutes. For topical use, dilute eucalyptus oil with a carrier oil (like coconut or olive oil) and apply to the chest or back 2–3 times a day.

Mullein (*Verbascum thapsus*)

Mullein is a powerful herb known for its ability to soothe and heal the respiratory tract. It is particularly effective for easing dry coughs, reducing inflammation, and expelling mucus from the lungs. Mullein has both expectorant and anti-inflammatory properties, making it ideal for conditions like bronchitis, asthma, and pneumonia. It also acts as a mild sedative, helping to calm the coughing reflex.

- **How to Use**: Mullein can be consumed as a tea, tincture, or capsule. The leaves and flowers are used in teas, while the tincture is more concentrated and can be taken in smaller doses.
- **Dosage**: For tea, steep 1–2 teaspoons of dried mullein flowers in hot water for 10–15 minutes, and drink 1–2 cups daily. For tincture, take 20–30 drops 2–3 times a day.

Licorice Root (*Glycyrrhiza glabra*)

Licorice root is a well-known herb with soothing, anti-inflammatory, and expectorant properties that can help relieve sore throats, coughs, and respiratory inflammation. It has been used for centuries in traditional medicine to treat bronchitis, asthma, and other lung issues. Licorice root helps to loosen mucus in the lungs, making it easier to cough up and clear the airways. It also supports the immune system and can fight off respiratory infections.

- **How to Use:** Licorice root is commonly consumed as a tea, tincture, or in capsules. It is also available in lozenge form to soothe the throat.
- **Dosage:** For tea, steep 1 teaspoon of dried licorice root in hot water for 5–10 minutes, and drink 1–2 cups daily. For tincture, take 10–20 drops 2–3 times a day. Be cautious with prolonged use, as licorice can affect blood pressure.

Thyme (*Thymus vulgaris*)

Thyme is a powerful herb with antimicrobial and expectorant properties that are excellent for supporting the respiratory system. It is particularly effective for treating coughs, bronchitis, and respiratory infections. Thyme helps to clear mucus from the airways, relax the muscles of the respiratory tract, and soothe the throat. Its high levels of antioxidants and flavonoids also support overall lung health and fight off infections.

- **How to Use:** Thyme can be consumed as a tea or used as a steam inhalant. The fresh or dried leaves can be brewed into a potent herbal tea, or essential oil can be inhaled to clear the airways.
- **Dosage:** For tea, use 1–2 teaspoons of dried thyme leaves per cup of hot water, and steep for 10–15 minutes. Drink 1–2 cups per day. For steam inhalation, add 2–3 drops of thyme essential oil to hot water and inhale the steam for 5–10 minutes.

Peppermint (*Mentha piperita*)

Peppermint is well-known for its refreshing aroma and cooling sensation, but it also offers significant respiratory benefits. The menthol in peppermint acts as a natural decongestant, helping to open the airways, reduce nasal congestion, and relieve coughing. Peppermint also has antispasmodic properties, making it useful for soothing the muscles of the respiratory tract and reducing the severity of asthma symptoms.

- **How to Use:** Peppermint can be consumed as a tea, used in steam inhalation, or applied topically in diluted oil form for chest congestion.
- **Dosage:** For tea, steep 1–2 teaspoons of dried peppermint leaves in hot water for 5–10 minutes, and drink 1–2 cups daily. For steam inhalation, add 2–3 drops of peppermint essential oil to hot water and inhale deeply. Topical application can be done with 1–2 drops of peppermint oil mixed with a carrier oil on the chest or neck.

Echinacea (*Echinacea purpurea*)

Echinacea is a well-known immune-boosting herb that also supports respiratory health. It is particularly effective for preventing and treating the common cold, flu, and upper respiratory infections. Echinacea has anti-inflammatory and antimicrobial properties, which help to reduce the severity and duration of respiratory infections. It also helps to strengthen the body's defense mechanisms against pathogens.

- **How to Use**: Echinacea is most commonly consumed as a tincture, tea, or capsule. It is typically used at the onset of a cold or respiratory infection to help reduce symptoms and speed recovery.
- **Dosage**: For tinctures, take 20–30 drops of echinacea extract 2–3 times a day. For tea, steep 1–2 teaspoons of dried echinacea root in hot water for 5–10 minutes and drink 1–2 cups daily. Capsules typically contain 300–500 mg, taken 1–2 times per day.

Osha Root (*Ligusticum porteri*)

Osha root is a potent herb traditionally used by Native Americans for respiratory health. It is particularly effective for relieving congestion, improving circulation in the lungs, and treating respiratory infections. Osha is known for its ability to soothe the respiratory tract, reduce inflammation, and enhance the body's ability to fight off infections. It is especially beneficial for chronic coughs, bronchitis, and sinusitis.

- **How to Use**: Osha root is typically consumed as a tincture, tea, or capsule. It is often used in combination with other respiratory herbs for enhanced effects.
- **Dosage**: For tincture, take 20–30 drops 2–3 times daily. For tea, steep 1 teaspoon of dried osha root in hot water for 10–15 minutes. Capsules typically contain 300–500 mg, taken 1–2 times per day.

Nettle (*Urtica dioica*)

Nettle is a versatile herb that offers numerous health benefits, including for respiratory health. It has natural antihistamine properties, which can help alleviate symptoms of allergies and hay fever, such as sneezing, runny nose, and itchy eyes. Nettle also supports overall lung health by reducing inflammation and promoting detoxification, making it useful for those with asthma or chronic respiratory issues.

- **How to Use**: Nettle is typically consumed as a tea or in capsule form. The leaves can be brewed into a mild tea that is both soothing and effective for respiratory support.
- **Dosage**: For tea, steep 1–2 teaspoons of dried nettle leaves in hot water for 10–15 minutes. Drink 1–2 cups daily. Capsules typically contain 300–500 mg, taken once or twice a day.

Liver and Detoxification Herbs

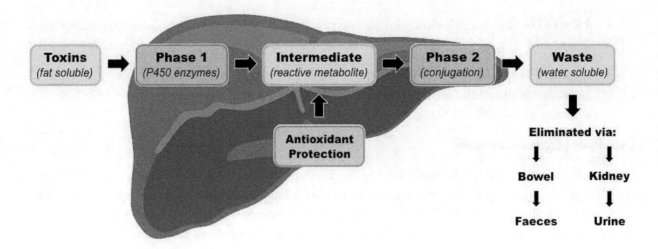

The liver plays a central role in detoxifying the body by filtering harmful substances from the blood, metabolizing nutrients, and producing bile to aid in digestion. However, due to factors such as poor diet, environmental toxins, stress, and excessive alcohol or medication use, the liver can become overburdened. When this happens, the body's natural detoxification process can slow down, leading to a range of issues such as fatigue, poor digestion, skin problems, and a weakened immune system.

Fortunately, nature offers a variety of herbs that support the liver's detoxification functions, promote healthy liver function, and help the body cleanse itself of toxins. These herbs are packed with antioxidants, flavonoids, and bioactive compounds that can protect the liver from damage, reduce inflammation, and enhance its ability to detoxify. Whether you're looking to improve liver health, support detoxification, or restore balance to your body, these herbs can be a valuable addition to your wellness routine.

Milk Thistle (*Silybum marianum*)

Milk thistle is perhaps the most well-known herb for liver health, thanks to its active compound, **silymarin**, which has powerful antioxidant and anti-inflammatory properties. Silymarin protects liver cells from toxins, supports liver regeneration, and helps detoxify harmful substances. Studies have shown that milk thistle can improve liver function in individuals with conditions such as fatty liver disease, hepatitis, and cirrhosis. It also aids in the digestion of fats by stimulating bile production.

- **How to Use:** Milk thistle is most commonly consumed as a standardized extract, tea, or capsule. The seeds contain the highest concentration of silymarin and are typically used in supplements.
- **Dosage:** A typical dosage is 200–400 mg of standardized milk thistle extract (containing 70–80% silymarin) taken 1–3 times per day. For tea, steep 1–2 teaspoons of dried milk thistle seeds in hot water for 5–10 minutes.

Dandelion Root (*Taraxacum officinale*)

Dandelion root is a gentle yet effective herb for promoting liver health and supporting detoxification. It acts as a natural diuretic, helping the body eliminate excess water and toxins. Dandelion root stimulates bile production, improving digestion and fat metabolism. It also has anti-inflammatory properties that support the liver and protect it from oxidative stress and damage. Regular use of dandelion root can help improve liver function and assist in detoxification.

- **How to Use:** Dandelion root can be consumed as a tea, tincture, or in capsule form. The root is often roasted for a more mild, earthy taste in teas.
- **Dosage:** For tea, steep 1–2 teaspoons of dried dandelion root in hot water for 10–15 minutes, and drink 1–2 cups daily. For tinctures, take 20–30 drops 2–3 times a day.

Burdock Root (*Arctium lappa*)

Burdock root is a powerful detoxifying herb known for its ability to support the liver and purify the blood. It is a natural diuretic and promotes the elimination of toxins through both the kidneys and liver. Burdock root also has antioxidant and anti-inflammatory properties that help protect the liver from damage while promoting the breakdown and removal of harmful substances. It is particularly helpful for improving skin conditions, such as acne or eczema, which can result from toxin buildup.

- **How to Use:** Burdock root can be consumed as a tea, tincture, or in capsule form. It is also commonly used in detox blends or as a part of liver-supporting herbal formulas.
- **Dosage:** For tea, use 1–2 teaspoons of dried burdock root in hot water, steeped for 10–15 minutes. Drink 1–2 cups daily. For tincture, take 20–30 drops 2–3 times per day.

Artichoke (*Cynara scolymus*)

Artichoke is not only a delicious vegetable but also a potent herb for supporting liver function and detoxification. Artichoke leaf extract has been shown to increase bile production, which helps the liver break down fats and detoxify more efficiently. It also supports liver cell regeneration and promotes the elimination of toxins from the bloodstream. Artichoke is particularly useful for those dealing with digestive issues related to liver function, such as bloating, indigestion, or gallbladder problems.

- **How to Use:** Artichoke is available in capsules, tablets, and liquid extracts. You can also consume the vegetable itself, which contains beneficial compounds for liver health.
- **Dosage:** For capsules or tablets, the typical dosage is 300–500 mg of artichoke extract, taken 1–2 times per day. For liquid extract, take 30–60 drops 2–3 times daily.

Turmeric (*Curcuma longa*)

Turmeric, specifically its active compound **curcumin**, is a powerful anti-inflammatory and antioxidant herb that offers significant support for liver health and detoxification. Curcumin helps protect the liver from damage caused by free radicals, reduces inflammation, and supports bile production. It also promotes the detoxification of heavy metals and other toxins from the liver. Additionally, turmeric has been shown to improve liver function in individuals with conditions like fatty liver disease and cirrhosis.

- **How to Use:** Turmeric can be consumed as a spice in food, as a supplement in capsule form, or as a tea. Curcumin is poorly absorbed on its own, so it's best consumed with black pepper or fat for improved bioavailability.

- **Dosage:** The typical dosage of turmeric or curcumin extract is 500–1000 mg per day. If using turmeric powder, 1–2 teaspoons can be added to warm water, milk, or smoothies. For turmeric tea, steep 1 teaspoon of turmeric root powder in hot water for 5–10 minutes.

Schisandra (*Schisandra chinensis*)

Schisandra, a potent adaptogenic herb, has long been used in Traditional Chinese Medicine (TCM) for its liver-supporting and detoxifying properties. Known as the "five-flavor fruit" due to its combination of sweet, sour, salty, bitter, and pungent tastes, schisandra helps protect liver cells from damage and supports the liver's ability to detoxify. It also promotes liver regeneration and increases antioxidant activity within the liver, which helps protect against oxidative stress.

- **How to Use:** Schisandra is most commonly consumed as a tincture, powder, or capsule. It can also be used to make tea, although the taste is quite unique and intense.

- **Dosage:** For tinctures, take 30–60 drops 2–3 times daily. For capsules, 500 mg is typically taken 1–2 times per day. If using powder, 1–2 teaspoons can be added to smoothies or teas.

Red Clover (*Trifolium pratense*)

Red clover is a natural blood purifier that supports liver health and detoxification. It helps cleanse the blood by promoting the elimination of toxins and supporting the lymphatic system. Red clover is rich in isoflavones, which have antioxidant properties that help reduce oxidative stress in the liver. This herb is often used in detox programs to support the body's ability to eliminate waste and promote overall liver health.

- **How to Use:** Red clover can be consumed as a tea, tincture, or in capsule form. The tea is mild and pleasant to drink, making it a popular option for daily liver support.

- **Dosage:** For tea, use 1–2 teaspoons of dried red clover flowers in hot water, steeped for 5–10 minutes. Drink 1–2 cups daily. For tincture, take 20–30 drops 2–3 times per day.

Ginger (*Zingiber officinale*)

Ginger is a well-known herb for its digestive benefits, but it also plays a key role in supporting liver health and detoxification. Ginger promotes bile production, which aids in fat digestion and helps the liver process toxins. Its anti-inflammatory and antioxidant properties support liver function, reduce inflammation, and help prevent liver damage. Ginger is also an excellent herb for stimulating circulation, further assisting the liver in its detoxification process.

- **How to Use:** Ginger can be consumed as fresh root, dried powder, or in supplement form. It is also widely used to make teas and tonics for digestive and liver support.

- **Dosage:** For fresh ginger root, 1–2 teaspoons of grated ginger can be added to hot water for tea. For powdered ginger, 1/2 teaspoon can be taken with warm water or added to smoothies. For supplements, 500–1000 mg of ginger extract is typically taken daily.

Cardiovascular Health Herbs

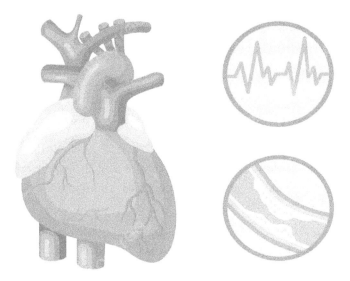

A healthy cardiovascular system is essential for overall well-being, as it ensures the effective circulation of blood, oxygen, and nutrients throughout the body. With heart disease being one of the leading causes of illness and death worldwide, maintaining cardiovascular health is a top priority for many. Fortunately, nature offers a variety of herbs that can support heart function, improve circulation, reduce blood pressure, and promote healthy cholesterol levels.

Cardiovascular health herbs contain bioactive compounds that help reduce inflammation, support blood vessel integrity, and regulate blood lipid levels. These herbs can be used as part of a holistic approach to heart health, alongside a balanced diet, regular exercise, and stress management. Whether you're looking to support overall heart function or address specific concerns such as high blood pressure or high cholesterol, the following herbs can play an important role in maintaining a healthy cardiovascular system.

Hawthorn (*Crataegus spp.*)

Hawthorn is one of the most widely used herbs for cardiovascular health, particularly for its ability to strengthen the heart, improve circulation, and regulate blood pressure. The berries, leaves, and flowers of the hawthorn plant contain flavonoids, antioxidants, and proanthocyanidins that help improve blood flow, reduce inflammation, and protect the heart from oxidative stress. Hawthorn is often used to support individuals with heart failure, irregular heart rhythms, and high blood pressure.

- **How to Use**: Hawthorn can be taken in the form of tea, tincture, or capsules. The berries and leaves are most commonly used for medicinal purposes.
- **Dosage**: For tea, steep 1–2 teaspoons of dried hawthorn berries or leaves in hot water for 10–15 minutes. Drink 1–2 cups daily. For tincture, take 20–30 drops 2–3 times per day. Capsules typically contain 250–500 mg of hawthorn extract, taken 1–2 times daily.

Garlic (*Allium sativum*)

Garlic is well-known for its many health benefits, and its positive impact on cardiovascular health is one of the most widely researched. Garlic contains sulfur compounds, such as allicin, which have been shown to lower blood pressure, reduce cholesterol levels, and improve overall heart health. Regular consumption of garlic can help prevent atherosclerosis (plaque buildup in the arteries), lower bad LDL cholesterol, and improve circulation.

- **How to Use:** Garlic can be consumed raw, in cooked dishes, or in supplement form. Garlic supplements are often available in odorless capsules, which provide the benefits without the strong smell.
- **Dosage:** To receive the cardiovascular benefits, aim for 1–2 cloves of fresh garlic daily. If using garlic supplements, 300–1,000 mg of aged garlic extract is a common daily dosage.

Ginger (*Zingiber officinale*)

Ginger is a powerful herb known for its anti-inflammatory and antioxidant properties, which make it beneficial for cardiovascular health. Ginger helps improve circulation, lower blood pressure, and reduce cholesterol levels. It also prevents the aggregation of platelets in the blood, which can help reduce the risk of blood clots. Regular use of ginger can improve blood vessel function and promote better overall heart health.

- **How to Use:** Ginger can be consumed fresh, in dried form, or as a supplement. It is commonly used in teas, smoothies, and cooking.
- **Dosage:** For tea, grate 1 teaspoon of fresh ginger and steep it in hot water for 5–10 minutes. Drink 1–2 cups daily. If using ginger supplements, 500–1,000 mg of ginger extract can be taken daily in divided doses.

Turmeric (*Curcuma longa*)

Turmeric is a golden-yellow root that contains the active compound curcumin, which is well-known for its powerful anti-inflammatory and antioxidant properties. Curcumin has been shown to benefit cardiovascular health by reducing inflammation, lowering cholesterol levels, and improving endothelial function (the health of blood vessels). It also helps prevent oxidative stress and the buildup of plaque in the arteries, reducing the risk of heart disease.

- **How to Use:** Turmeric can be added to food, taken as a supplement, or brewed into tea. To enhance absorption, it is often combined with black pepper (which contains piperine, a compound that increases curcumin absorption) or healthy fats like coconut oil.
- **Dosage:** For turmeric powder, 1–2 teaspoons can be added to warm milk, smoothies, or soups. Curcumin supplements typically range from 500–1,000 mg per day, taken with black pepper for optimal absorption.

Coenzyme Q10 (CoQ10)

Coenzyme Q10, or CoQ10, is a naturally occurring antioxidant found in every cell of the body, especially in the heart. It plays a crucial role in energy production within cells and helps protect the heart from oxidative damage. CoQ10 has been shown to lower blood pressure, improve blood vessel function, and reduce the risk of heart disease. It is particularly beneficial for individuals taking statins, as these medications can deplete natural CoQ10 levels in the body.

- **How to Use:** CoQ10 is available in supplement form as capsules or soft gels. It can also be found in certain foods, such as organ meats, oily fish, and whole grains, though supplementation is often more effective for therapeutic purposes.
- **Dosage:** The typical dosage for CoQ10 is 100–200 mg per day, though some individuals may take up to 400 mg daily under the guidance of a healthcare provider.

Cayenne Pepper (*Capsicum annuum*)

Cayenne pepper, which contains the active compound capsaicin, has a stimulating effect on circulation and heart health. Capsaicin promotes blood flow by relaxing blood vessels, which helps lower blood pressure and reduce the risk of heart disease. It also supports fat metabolism and helps to maintain a healthy weight, further contributing to overall cardiovascular health.

- **How to Use:** Cayenne pepper can be added to food or taken in supplement form. It can also be used to make spicy herbal teas.
- **Dosage:** A typical dosage of cayenne pepper is 1/4 to 1/2 teaspoon of powdered cayenne added to food or tea. If using cayenne supplements, start with 30–120 mg of capsaicin daily.

Flaxseed (*Linum usitatissimum*)

Flaxseed is rich in omega-3 fatty acids, fiber, and lignans, all of which contribute to heart health. The omega-3s in flaxseed help reduce inflammation, lower triglyceride levels, and improve cholesterol balance by raising HDL ("good") cholesterol and lowering LDL ("bad") cholesterol. Flaxseed also supports healthy blood pressure levels by improving blood vessel function and reducing oxidative stress.

- **How to Use:** Flaxseed can be consumed as whole seeds, ground flaxseed, or in oil form. Ground flaxseed is the most effective way to absorb its nutrients.
- **Dosage:** A typical daily dosage is 1–2 tablespoons of ground flaxseed or 1–2 teaspoons of flaxseed oil. If using flaxseed oil supplements, 1,000–2,000 mg per day is recommended.

Cinnamon (*Cinnamomum verum*)

Cinnamon is a delicious spice that has long been used for its health benefits, including its positive effects on cardiovascular health. Cinnamon helps regulate blood sugar levels, reduce cholesterol, and improve circulation. The active compound **cinnamaldehyde** in cinnamon has been shown to reduce inflammation in the arteries and protect the heart from oxidative damage.

- **How to Use:** Cinnamon can be added to food, smoothies, or teas. Ceylon cinnamon (often referred to as "true cinnamon") is preferred over cassia cinnamon for health benefits, as it contains lower levels of coumarin, which can be harmful in large amounts.
- **Dosage:** A typical dosage of cinnamon powder is 1/2 to 1 teaspoon daily. For cinnamon supplements, the usual dosage is 500–1,000 mg per day.

Ashwagandha (*Withania somnifera*)

Ashwagandha is an adaptogenic herb that helps the body cope with stress, which is an important factor in cardiovascular health. Chronic stress contributes to high blood pressure, heart disease, and other cardiovascular conditions. Ashwagandha helps lower cortisol levels, reduce anxiety, and improve overall heart function. It is also thought to support healthy blood sugar levels, which indirectly supports cardiovascular health.

- **How to Use:** Ashwagandha is available in powder, capsule, and liquid extract forms. It can be taken with warm milk, water, or added to smoothies.

- **Dosage:** The typical dosage of ashwagandha root extract is 300–500 mg, taken once or twice a day. The powder form can be taken in doses of 1–2 teaspoons daily.

Hormonal Health Herbs

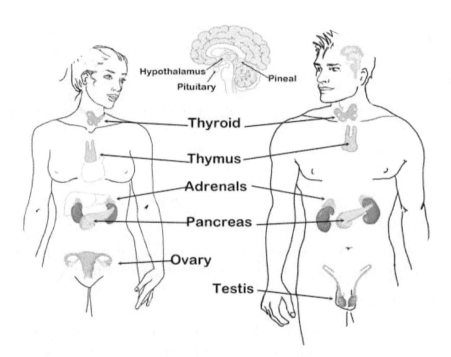

Hormones are chemical messengers that regulate various processes in the body, including metabolism, mood, energy, reproduction, and immune function. When hormones are balanced, the body functions optimally; however, hormonal imbalances can lead to a wide range of symptoms and health concerns, including fatigue, weight gain or loss, mood swings, irregular menstrual cycles, and diminished libido. Factors such as stress, poor diet, environmental toxins, aging, and certain medical conditions can disrupt hormonal balance.

Fortunately, herbal medicine offers a natural and holistic approach to supporting hormonal health. Many herbs contain bioactive compounds that can help regulate hormone production, support the endocrine system, and alleviate symptoms associated with hormonal imbalances. These herbs are particularly helpful for conditions like PMS (premenstrual syndrome), menopause, thyroid imbalances, and adrenal fatigue.

Ashwagandha (*Withania somnifera*)

Ashwagandha is an adaptogenic herb renowned for its ability to help the body cope with stress, which is a major factor in hormonal imbalances. Chronic stress increases the production of cortisol, a stress hormone that can disrupt the balance of other hormones, including thyroid hormones and sex hormones. Ashwagandha works to reduce cortisol levels, support adrenal function, and enhance overall hormonal balance. Additionally, it is known to improve thyroid function and support reproductive health by stabilizing estrogen and progesterone levels.

- **How to Use**: Ashwagandha is available in powder, capsule, and liquid extract forms. The powder can be mixed with warm milk, water, or smoothies.
- **Dosage**: The typical dosage is 300–500 mg of standardized ashwagandha extract per day, taken in one or two doses. For powder, 1–2 teaspoons daily are recommended.

Vitex (Chaste Tree Berry) (*Vitex agnus-castus*)

Vitex, also known as chaste tree berry, is a highly regarded herb for balancing female hormones. It has a long history of use in treating menstrual disorders, including PMS, irregular cycles, and menopause symptoms. Vitex works by stimulating the pituitary gland, which in turn helps regulate the production of progesterone and estrogen. By promoting hormonal balance, Vitex can help alleviate symptoms such as mood swings, breast tenderness, and irregular menstruation.

- **How to Use**: Vitex is commonly used as a tincture, capsule, or tea. It can also be found in combination with other herbs designed for female health.
- **Dosage**: For tincture, 20–30 drops can be taken 2–3 times daily. The typical dosage for capsules is 400–500 mg per day, taken once daily, preferably in the morning.

Black Cohosh (*Actaea racemosa*)

Black cohosh is a well-known herb used primarily to address symptoms related to menopause, including hot flashes, night sweats, mood swings, and vaginal dryness. It is thought to work by influencing estrogen receptors in the body, thus alleviating common menopausal symptoms without introducing synthetic hormones. Black cohosh also supports the nervous system and helps manage the emotional fluctuations often associated with hormonal shifts during menopause.

- **How to Use**: Black cohosh is typically consumed as a capsule, tablet, or tincture. It is often combined with other herbs to enhance its effects during menopause.
- **Dosage**: For menopause-related symptoms, 20–40 mg of black cohosh extract (standardized to 2.5% triterpene glycosides) can be taken once or twice daily. For tincture, 20–30 drops, 2–3 times per day, is common.

Maca Root (*Lepidium meyenii*)

Maca root is a powerful adaptogen that has been used for centuries to enhance energy, improve mood, and balance hormones. It is especially beneficial for women experiencing hormonal fluctuations due to menopause or PCOS (polycystic ovary syndrome). Maca helps to regulate the production of estrogen and progesterone, reduce symptoms of fatigue and low libido, and improve overall hormonal health. For men, maca is also known to support testosterone levels and improve fertility.

- **How to Use:** Maca root is available in powder, capsule, or liquid form. The powder can be added to smoothies, oatmeal, or other foods.
- **Dosage:** A typical dosage is 1,500–3,000 mg of maca root powder daily, or 500–1,000 mg of maca extract in capsule form.

Red Clover (*Trifolium pratense*)

Red clover is a rich source of phytoestrogens—plant compounds that mimic the effects of estrogen in the body. As a result, red clover is particularly useful for women going through menopause or experiencing symptoms related to low estrogen levels. It can help reduce hot flashes, improve bone health, and support cardiovascular function. Red clover is also beneficial for women with irregular periods or hormonal acne, as it promotes overall hormonal balance.

- **How to Use:** Red clover can be consumed as a tea, tincture, or in capsules.
- **Dosage:** For tea, steep 1–2 teaspoons of dried red clover flowers in hot water for 5–10 minutes. Drink 1–2 cups per day. For tincture, 20–30 drops, 2–3 times a day, is common.

Dong Quai (*Angelica sinensis*)

Dong Quai, often referred to as the "female ginseng," is a traditional herb used in Chinese medicine to support female reproductive health. It is especially helpful for addressing symptoms of hormonal imbalance, such as irregular menstruation, PMS, and menopause. Dong Quai works by nourishing and regulating the blood, enhancing circulation, and promoting the balance of estrogen levels. It is also known to improve mood and alleviate the fatigue often associated with hormonal changes.

- **How to Use:** Dong Quai is available in capsule, tincture, or tea form.
- **Dosage:** The typical dosage for Dong Quai capsules is 500–1,000 mg per day, taken in divided doses. For tinctures, 20–30 drops, 2–3 times daily, is standard.

Shatavari (*Asparagus racemosus*)

Shatavari is a well-known herb in Ayurvedic medicine for supporting female reproductive health and hormonal balance. It is especially beneficial for women experiencing fertility issues, menstrual irregularities, or menopausal symptoms. Shatavari helps regulate estrogen levels, improve ovarian health, and enhance the body's ability to manage stress, which can be a significant factor in hormonal imbalances. It is often referred to as a "female tonic" due to its supportive effects on overall reproductive health.

- **How to Use:** Shatavari is typically available in powder, capsule, or liquid extract form. It is commonly consumed with warm milk or water.

- **Dosage**: For powder, 1–2 teaspoons can be taken with warm milk or water, 1–2 times per day. In capsule form, 500–1,000 mg per day is recommended.

Tribulus Terrestris (*Tribulus terrestris*)

Tribulus Terrestris is an herb widely used for its ability to support reproductive health and hormone balance, particularly in men and women with low libido. It has been shown to enhance the production of luteinizing hormone (LH), which in turn stimulates the production of estrogen in women and testosterone in men. Tribulus is also used to improve fertility, increase libido, and promote better sexual health.

- **How to Use**: Tribulus Terrestris is available in capsules, tablets, and tinctures.
- **Dosage**: A typical dosage is 250–500 mg of Tribulus extract taken once or twice per day.

Evening Primrose Oil (*Oenothera biennis*)

Evening primrose oil is rich in gamma-linolenic acid (GLA), an essential fatty acid that plays a key role in hormone production and regulation. GLA supports the body's ability to produce prostaglandins, which are involved in the regulation of menstrual cycles, inflammation, and immune function. Evening primrose oil is especially helpful for women with PMS, as it can reduce symptoms such as breast tenderness, mood swings, and irritability. It also helps balance estrogen levels during menopause.

- **How to Use**: Evening primrose oil is most commonly consumed in capsule or softgel form.
- **Dosage**: The typical dosage is 500–1,000 mg of evening primrose oil per day, taken in divided doses.

Blood Sugar & Weight Management Herbs

Maintaining balanced blood sugar levels and managing a healthy weight are crucial for overall health. Imbalances in blood sugar can lead to conditions like insulin resistance, type 2 diabetes, and metabolic syndrome, while weight management is often a challenge for those dealing with these conditions or struggling with excess weight. Fortunately, nature offers a wide range of herbs that can support both blood sugar regulation and weight management, promoting long-term wellness without the need for synthetic interventions.

Herbal remedies for blood sugar and weight management often work through different mechanisms, including improving insulin sensitivity, reducing blood sugar spikes, enhancing fat metabolism, and controlling appetite. Incorporating these herbs into a holistic lifestyle, which includes proper diet, regular physical activity, and stress management, can significantly enhance your health outcomes.

Cinnamon (*Cinnamomum verum*)

Cinnamon is a widely used spice that not only adds flavor to dishes but also offers impressive health benefits, particularly for blood sugar regulation. Studies have shown that cinnamon can enhance insulin sensitivity, allowing the body to use glucose more efficiently. This helps to lower blood sugar levels and prevent spikes after meals. Additionally, cinnamon may reduce fasting blood sugar levels and improve lipid profiles, making it beneficial for people with type 2 diabetes and those trying to manage their weight.

- **How to Use:** Cinnamon can be added to smoothies, oatmeal, baked goods, or brewed as tea. It's also available in capsule and powder form.
- **Dosage:** A typical dosage is 1/2 to 1 teaspoon of ground cinnamon per day, either as a powder in food or beverages. If using cinnamon supplements, 500–1,000 mg per day is common.

Gymnema Sylvestre (*Gymnema sylvestre*)

Known as the "sugar destroyer" in traditional herbal medicine, **Gymnema Sylvestre** has been used for centuries to help control blood sugar levels. The active compounds in Gymnema can block sugar receptors in the intestines, reducing the absorption of sugar and lowering blood glucose levels. Additionally, Gymnema has been shown to stimulate insulin production and improve insulin sensitivity. It's particularly helpful for individuals with type 2 diabetes and those who want to curb sugar cravings.

- **How to Use:** Gymnema is typically consumed as a capsule, tablet, or tincture. It is also available as a tea.
- **Dosage:** Standard dosages range from 200–400 mg of Gymnema extract per day, taken in divided doses. For tea, 1–2 teaspoons of dried Gymnema leaves can be steeped in hot water for 10–15 minutes.

Bitter Melon (*Momordica charantia*)

Bitter melon is a fruit that has long been used in traditional medicine to help manage blood sugar levels. It contains compounds that mimic insulin, which helps to lower blood glucose by improving glucose uptake into cells. Bitter melon has also been shown to improve lipid profiles, reduce insulin resistance, and support weight loss by promoting fat metabolism. It can be especially helpful for those with type 2 diabetes and those struggling with obesity.

- **How to Use:** Bitter melon can be consumed as a juice, in stir-fries, or taken as a supplement in capsule or powder form. It is also available as a tea.
- **Dosage:** The typical dosage is 500–1,000 mg of bitter melon extract daily, or 1–2 teaspoons of the powdered form. For bitter melon tea, 1 teaspoon of dried fruit is steeped in hot water for 10 minutes.

Fenugreek (*Trigonella foenum-graecum*)

Fenugreek is an herb that has gained popularity for its ability to regulate blood sugar levels and aid in weight management. Fenugreek seeds contain soluble fiber, which slows down the absorption of sugar in the digestive tract, preventing blood sugar spikes. They also contain compounds that enhance insulin sensitivity, helping the body utilize glucose more effectively. Additionally, fenugreek has appetite-suppressing properties, which can help reduce overeating and promote weight loss.

- **How to Use:** Fenugreek can be consumed as seeds, powder, or in supplement form. Fenugreek tea is also a common way to use this herb.

- **Dosage**: A common dosage is 1–2 teaspoons of fenugreek seeds daily, or 500–1,000 mg of fenugreek extract. For tea, steep 1 teaspoon of seeds in hot water for 5–10 minutes.

Berberine (*Berberis vulgaris*)

Berberine is a potent plant compound found in several herbs, including **golden seal** and **barberry**. It has been extensively researched for its ability to regulate blood sugar, improve insulin sensitivity, and promote weight loss. Berberine works by activating an enzyme called AMP-activated protein kinase (AMPK), which plays a crucial role in regulating metabolism, glucose uptake, and fat breakdown. Berberine has been shown to reduce blood sugar levels and improve metabolic function in individuals with type 2 diabetes.

- **How to Use**: Berberine is commonly available in supplement form as capsules or tablets. It is not typically consumed in food or drink.
- **Dosage**: The typical dosage is 500 mg of berberine, taken 2–3 times per day before meals. It's important to start with a lower dose and gradually increase it to minimize gastrointestinal discomfort.

Turmeric (*Curcuma longa*)

Turmeric, particularly its active compound curcumin, has long been valued for its anti-inflammatory and antioxidant properties. Research suggests that curcumin can help reduce inflammation in the body, which plays a key role in insulin resistance and weight gain. Additionally, turmeric may help regulate blood sugar levels and promote fat metabolism. It also supports the healthy function of the liver, which is crucial for overall metabolic health.

- **How to Use**: Turmeric can be consumed as a spice in cooking, in smoothies, or as a tea. It is also available in supplement form as capsules or tablets.
- **Dosage**: A common dosage of turmeric is 500–1,000 mg of curcumin extract per day, often taken with black pepper (which enhances curcumin absorption). If using turmeric powder, 1–2 teaspoons per day is typical.

Ginger (*Zingiber officinale*)

Ginger is not only a popular culinary herb but also a powerful tool for supporting healthy blood sugar levels and promoting weight loss. Ginger has been shown to improve insulin sensitivity, reduce fasting blood glucose levels, and decrease inflammation. Additionally, ginger can aid digestion, reduce bloating, and enhance fat metabolism, making it beneficial for those trying to manage weight.

- **How to Use**: Ginger can be consumed fresh, dried, or in supplement form. It is commonly used in teas, smoothies, and cooking.
- **Dosage**: For tea, 1–2 teaspoons of grated fresh ginger can be steeped in hot water for 5–10 minutes. Ginger supplements typically contain 500–1,000 mg per dose, taken 1–2 times daily.

Clove (*Syzygium aromaticum*)

Cloves are rich in antioxidants and have been shown to improve insulin sensitivity and support healthy blood sugar levels. They contain a compound called eugenol, which helps reduce oxidative stress and inflammation in the body, both of which can contribute to insulin resistance and weight gain. Cloves also help with digestion, reduce bloating, and support a healthy metabolism.

- **How to Use:** Cloves can be used in cooking, added to teas, or taken in powdered form. Clove oil and supplements are also available.
- **Dosage:** A typical dosage is 1–2 teaspoons of ground cloves per day, either added to food or brewed as tea. If using clove supplements, 500–1,000 mg per day is common.

Aloe Vera (*Aloe barbadensis miller*)

Aloe vera, widely known for its skin-soothing properties, also offers significant benefits for blood sugar regulation. Aloe vera can help lower fasting blood sugar levels, improve insulin sensitivity, and reduce inflammation in the body. Additionally, it supports digestive health, which can aid in the efficient absorption of nutrients and promote overall weight management.

- **How to Use:** Aloe vera can be consumed as a juice or in supplement form. The gel can also be added to smoothies.
- **Dosage:** Aloe vera juice should be consumed in small amounts (2–4 oz per day), or aloe vera supplements (typically 200–500 mg) can be taken daily.

Anti-inflammatory & Pain Relief Herbs

Inflammation is a natural response by the body to injury, infection, or stress. However, chronic inflammation can contribute to a variety of health issues, including joint pain, muscle soreness, arthritis, cardiovascular disease, and even autoimmune disorders. Inflammation often comes hand-in-hand with pain, which can affect daily life, making even simple tasks feel overwhelming. While pharmaceutical medications can offer relief, many people are turning to natural remedies to manage inflammation and pain with fewer side effects.

Herbs have been used for centuries for their ability to reduce inflammation and alleviate pain. These healing plants contain powerful bioactive compounds that target the underlying causes of pain and inflammation, helping to restore balance and promote healing without the risk of long-term side effects commonly associated with synthetic drugs. In this guide, we will explore some of the most effective herbs known for their anti-inflammatory and pain-relieving properties.

Turmeric (*Curcuma longa*)

Turmeric is one of the most well-known anti-inflammatory herbs, largely due to its active compound, **curcumin**. Curcumin is a potent antioxidant with powerful anti-inflammatory properties that has been shown to reduce the levels of pro-inflammatory cytokines and enzymes in the body, such as COX-2. By inhibiting these inflammatory compounds, turmeric can effectively reduce pain and swelling associated with conditions like arthritis, muscle soreness, and even chronic pain conditions.

- **How to Use**: Turmeric can be used fresh, dried, or as a powder in cooking, smoothies, and teas. It is also available in capsule or tablet form.

- **Dosage**: The typical dosage is 500–1,000 mg of curcumin extract per day, often taken with black pepper to enhance absorption. For fresh turmeric, 1–2 teaspoons of grated turmeric root can be used daily.

Ginger (*Zingiber officinale*)

Ginger is another herb with well-documented anti-inflammatory and analgesic (pain-relieving) properties. The active compounds in ginger, such as **gingerol** and **shogaol**, help reduce the production of inflammatory molecules and enzymes like COX-2. Studies have shown that ginger is effective for treating pain associated with osteoarthritis, rheumatoid arthritis, and muscle injuries. It is also commonly used to reduce nausea, improve digestion, and support overall immune function.

- **How to Use**: Fresh or dried ginger can be added to smoothies, teas, soups, or used as a spice in cooking. Ginger supplements are also widely available.

- **Dosage**: For fresh ginger, 1–2 teaspoons of grated ginger can be consumed daily. Ginger extract supplements typically range from 500–1,000 mg per day.

Boswellia (*Boswellia serrata*)

Boswellia, also known as **Indian frankincense**, is a tree resin with a long history of use in Ayurvedic medicine. Boswellia contains **boswellic acids**, which have potent anti-inflammatory effects that can help reduce pain and swelling, particularly in conditions like osteoarthritis, rheumatoid arthritis, and inflammatory bowel disease (IBD). Boswellia works by inhibiting the activity of 5-lipoxygenase, an enzyme responsible for producing inflammatory compounds, thereby reducing both inflammation and pain.

- **How to Use**: Boswellia is commonly found in capsule or tablet form. It can also be taken as a tincture or extract.

- **Dosage**: A typical dosage is 300–500 mg of standardized Boswellia extract (containing 60% boswellic acids) taken 2–3 times per day.

White Willow Bark (*Salix alba*)

White willow bark has been used for centuries as a natural pain reliever and anti-inflammatory agent. The bark contains **salicin**, a compound that is chemically similar to aspirin. Once ingested, the body converts salicin into salicylic acid, which helps to reduce pain, inflammation, and fever. White willow bark is particularly useful for treating chronic pain conditions like back pain, osteoarthritis, and headaches, as well as for reducing overall muscle soreness and inflammation.

- **How to Use**: White willow bark is available in capsule, tablet, or tincture form. It can also be brewed into a tea.

- **Dosage**: The typical dosage is 60–120 mg of salicin per day, or 1–2 teaspoons of dried bark brewed in water to make tea. If using a tincture, 1–2 ml, 2–3 times per day, is common.

Arnica (*Arnica montana*)

Arnica is a powerful herb known for its ability to reduce pain, swelling, and bruising. It is most commonly used topically as a cream, gel, or ointment for treating muscle aches, sprains, bruises, and joint pain. Arnica works by stimulating blood flow to the affected area and reducing inflammation, making it effective for both acute injuries and chronic pain conditions.

- **How to Use:** Arnica is available as a topical cream, gel, or ointment, and can be applied directly to the skin over sore or inflamed areas. It is also available in homeopathic form.
- **Dosage:** For topical use, apply a thin layer of arnica gel or cream to the affected area 2–3 times per day. For homeopathic preparations, follow the instructions provided on the label.

Capsaicin (*Capsicum annuum*)

Capsaicin is the active compound found in chili peppers and is widely used in topical creams for pain relief. Capsaicin works by desensitizing the sensory nerve fibers in the skin, reducing the sensation of pain over time. It is particularly effective for treating conditions like neuropathic pain, arthritis, and muscle pain, and has been shown to reduce pain signals sent to the brain.

- **How to Use:** Capsaicin is typically found in topical creams, ointments, or patches. It can be applied directly to the skin.
- **Dosage:** Apply a thin layer of capsaicin cream (typically containing 0.025–0.075% capsaicin) to the affected area 2–3 times per day. Avoid contact with eyes or broken skin.

Devil's Claw (*Harpagophytum procumbens*)

Devil's Claw is a herb native to southern Africa that has been traditionally used to treat pain and inflammation. The active compounds in devil's claw, primarily **harpagoside**, have been shown to reduce inflammation and alleviate pain, particularly in cases of osteoarthritis, back pain, and muscle soreness. Devil's claw is believed to inhibit the production of pro-inflammatory cytokines and enzymes, making it a valuable herb for managing chronic pain.

- **How to Use:** Devil's claw is typically taken in capsule, tablet, or tincture form. It can also be brewed into tea.
- **Dosage:** A typical dosage of devil's claw extract is 600–1,200 mg per day, divided into two doses.

Lavender (*Lavandula angustifolia*)

Lavender is known for its calming effects on the nervous system, but it also has mild anti-inflammatory and analgesic properties. It is particularly useful for relieving tension headaches, migraines, and muscle pain, as well as promoting relaxation and sleep. Lavender can be used both topically and aromatically to reduce pain and inflammation.

- **How to Use:** Lavender essential oil can be used in a diffuser, added to a warm bath, or diluted with a carrier oil and massaged into the skin. Lavender tea is also commonly consumed.
- **Dosage:** For essential oil, add 3–5 drops to a diffuser or dilute with a carrier oil and apply to sore areas. For tea, steep 1 teaspoon of dried lavender flowers in hot water for 5–10 minutes.

Nettle (*Urtica dioica*)

Nettle is a nutrient-dense herb that has been used traditionally for its anti-inflammatory properties. It is particularly helpful for managing joint pain, especially in conditions like rheumatoid arthritis and osteoarthritis. Nettle contains compounds that reduce inflammation, support joint health, and promote the elimination of toxins from the body, helping to reduce pain and stiffness.

- **How to Use**: Nettle is available in capsule, tablet, and tincture forms. It can also be consumed as a tea.
- **Dosage**: For tea, steep 1–2 teaspoons of dried nettle leaves in hot water for 10–15 minutes. For capsules, 300–500 mg of nettle extract is commonly taken 2–3 times daily.

Antioxidant & Anti-Aging Herbs

As we age, our bodies undergo a variety of natural changes—many of which are linked to the cumulative effects of oxidative stress and cellular damage. Free radicals, unstable molecules generated by environmental factors, stress, and the natural aging process, can accelerate the breakdown of cells, tissues, and organs. Over time, this oxidative damage contributes to aging skin, wrinkles, sagging, and the decline of bodily functions. However, nature has equipped us with an array of herbs rich in antioxidants—compounds that neutralize these harmful free radicals and slow down the aging process.

Antioxidant and anti-aging herbs not only protect your cells from oxidative stress but also support overall health by boosting your immune system, promoting healthy skin, improving mental clarity, and enhancing energy levels. By incorporating these herbs into your wellness routine, you can effectively combat the visible and invisible signs of aging while supporting long-term vitality.

Ashwagandha (*Withania somnifera*)

Ashwagandha, often referred to as **Indian ginseng**, is an adaptogenic herb that has been used for centuries in Ayurvedic medicine. Known for its ability to reduce stress and support adrenal health, ashwagandha also possesses strong antioxidant properties. It helps reduce oxidative damage to cells, combats the effects of chronic stress, and supports the body's natural defenses. By regulating cortisol levels and reducing inflammation, ashwagandha not only helps to slow the aging process but also promotes energy, stamina, and mental clarity.

- **How to Use**: Ashwagandha is available in capsule, powder, or tincture form. It can also be added to smoothies or taken with warm milk or water.
- **Dosage**: A typical dosage is 300–500 mg of standardized extract, taken 1–2 times per day.

Green Tea (*Camellia sinensis*)

Green tea is a powerhouse of antioxidants, particularly **catechins** such as **epigallocatechin gallate (EGCG)**, which are well-known for their anti-aging effects. These antioxidants help neutralize free radicals, preventing premature skin aging and protecting the body from cellular damage. Green tea has also been shown to improve skin elasticity, reduce wrinkles, and increase skin hydration. Moreover, it supports cardiovascular health, boosts metabolism, and improves brain function, making it a comprehensive anti-aging herb.

- **How to Use:** Green tea can be consumed as a hot beverage, cold brew, or in supplement form (extracts or capsules).
- **Dosage:** Drink 2–3 cups of green tea per day, or take 300–400 mg of green tea extract in capsule form.

Ginseng (*Panax ginseng*)

Ginseng is an iconic herb used for centuries in traditional medicine, prized for its ability to promote longevity and enhance vitality. The active compounds in ginseng, particularly **ginsenosides**, are potent antioxidants that help protect cells from oxidative damage, reduce inflammation, and support cognitive function. By stimulating blood circulation and boosting energy levels, ginseng combats the fatigue and physical decline associated with aging, while improving skin tone and texture for a more youthful appearance.

- **How to Use:** Ginseng can be consumed as a tea, powder, or in capsules. It is also available as a tincture or extract.
- **Dosage:** The typical dosage is 200–400 mg of ginseng extract per day, or 1–2 teaspoons of powdered ginseng root.

Turmeric (*Curcuma longa*)

Turmeric, particularly its active compound **curcumin**, is widely celebrated for its potent antioxidant and anti-inflammatory properties. Curcumin neutralizes free radicals and enhances the body's own antioxidant enzymes, protecting the cells from damage and slowing the aging process. Regular use of turmeric has been shown to improve skin health by reducing fine lines, wrinkles, and hyperpigmentation. Furthermore, it supports joint health, cognitive function, and heart health, making it a holistic anti-aging herb.

- **How to Use:** Turmeric can be used in cooking, smoothies, or taken as a supplement in capsule or tablet form.
- **Dosage:** A typical dosage is 500–1,000 mg of curcumin extract per day, preferably taken with black pepper to enhance absorption.

Schisandra (*Schisandra chinensis*)

Schisandra, a berry-producing vine from traditional Chinese medicine, is known for its ability to promote youthful energy and vitality. This herb is classified as an adaptogen, meaning it helps the body adapt to stress while promoting balance and harmony. Schisandra is rich in **lignans**, powerful antioxidants that protect the liver, support skin health, and improve endurance. It also has the unique ability to enhance mental clarity, reduce fatigue, and support a healthy aging process by rejuvenating the body's energy systems.

- **How to Use:** Schisandra is available in powder, capsule, or tincture form. It can also be added to smoothies or teas.

- **Dosage:** The standard dosage is 500–1,000 mg of schisandra extract per day, or 1–2 teaspoons of powdered schisandra berries.

Gotu Kola (*Centella Asiatica*)

Gotu kola, often called the "herb of longevity," has been used in traditional medicine for centuries to promote healthy aging and cognitive function. It is rich in antioxidants and triterpenoids, which help stimulate collagen production and protect the skin from oxidative damage. Gotu kola supports healthy circulation, reduces the appearance of scars and stretch marks, and helps to heal wounds, making it particularly beneficial for skin health. It also enhances mental clarity and memory, making it an ideal herb for supporting both physical and cognitive longevity.

- **How to Use:** Gotu kola can be consumed as a tea, tincture, or in capsule form. It is also available as a topical cream or ointment for skin application.
- **Dosage:** The typical dosage is 500–1,000 mg of standardized extract, taken 1–2 times per day. For tea, steep 1–2 teaspoons of dried gotu kola leaves in hot water for 10 minutes.

Resveratrol (*Polygonum cuspidatum*)

Resveratrol is a polyphenolic compound found in the skin of red grapes, as well as in berries and peanuts. It is well-known for its antioxidant properties, which help protect cells from oxidative stress and support healthy aging. Resveratrol has been shown to activate **sirtuins**, enzymes that play a key role in regulating the aging process at the cellular level. By promoting healthy mitochondrial function and reducing inflammation, resveratrol supports cardiovascular health, protects the skin from UV damage, and may even promote longevity.

- **How to Use:** Resveratrol is commonly consumed as an extract in supplement form, although it can also be obtained from red wine and certain berries.
- **Dosage:** A typical dosage of resveratrol is 100–500 mg per day, taken in capsule or tablet form.

Bilberry (*Vaccinium myrtillus*)

Bilberries are rich in **anthocyanins**, a type of flavonoid that acts as a powerful antioxidant to protect cells from oxidative damage. These antioxidants have been shown to promote healthy vision, improve circulation, and support skin health by increasing collagen production and reducing signs of aging. Bilberries are particularly useful in improving skin elasticity, reducing fine lines, and providing protection from UV-induced skin aging. Additionally, they support brain health and cognitive function, making them a great herb for anti-aging.

- **How to Use:** Bilberries can be consumed fresh, dried, or in supplement form as capsules or extracts.
- **Dosage:** A typical dosage is 500–1,000 mg of bilberry extract per day, or 1–2 teaspoons of dried bilberries for tea.

Milk Thistle (*Silybum marianum*)

Milk thistle is widely known for its liver-protecting properties due to its active compound **silymarin**, which is a potent antioxidant. By protecting the liver from oxidative damage and supporting detoxification, milk thistle helps the body eliminate toxins that can accelerate aging. Additionally, milk thistle supports skin health, reducing wrinkles and promoting a glowing complexion by improving liver function and detoxification processes.

- **How to Use:** Milk thistle is available in capsule, tablet, or tincture form, and can also be brewed as a tea.
- **Dosage:** The typical dosage of milk thistle extract is 200–400 mg of silymarin per day, taken in divided doses.

Anti-Viral & Antibacterial Herbs

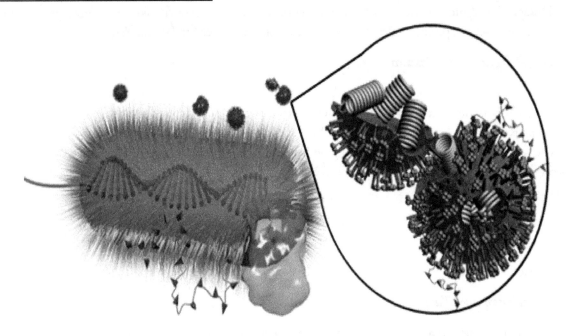

In our modern world, exposure to pathogens is nearly unavoidable, whether through air, food, or touch. From the common cold to more severe viral or bacterial infections, our immune systems face constant threats. While antibiotics and antiviral medications play a crucial role in combating infections, nature provides us with a wide range of herbs that have proven anti-viral and antibacterial properties. These herbs not only help to prevent and treat infections but also support the body's immune system, reduce inflammation, and promote faster healing.

Echinacea (*Echinacea purpurea*)

Echinacea is one of the most popular and widely used herbs for boosting immune function. It contains active compounds such as **echinacosides**, **polysaccharides**, and **flavonoids**, which enhance the body's immune response and help fight off infections. Studies suggest that Echinacea is particularly effective in preventing and shortening the duration of the common cold, and it also has antibacterial and antiviral properties that can support the body during a variety of infections, including respiratory illnesses.

- **How to Use**: Echinacea can be consumed as a tea, tincture, or in capsule or tablet form. It is also available as an extract.
- **Dosage**: For acute conditions, 300–500 mg of Echinacea extract is typically taken 2–3 times per day. If using as a preventive measure, 300–500 mg daily is sufficient.

Garlic (*Allium sativum*)

Garlic has long been revered for its powerful antibacterial, antiviral, and antifungal properties. The active compound in garlic, **allicin**, has been shown to fight infections by disrupting the cell membranes of bacteria and viruses, thereby preventing their replication. Garlic has a broad spectrum of activity and is effective against common cold viruses, influenza, and even certain bacterial strains, including antibiotic-resistant ones like **MRSA** (Methicillin-resistant Staphylococcus aureus). In addition to its antimicrobial properties, garlic boosts the immune system, reduces inflammation, and supports cardiovascular health.

- **How to Use**: Garlic can be consumed raw, crushed, or in supplement form. It can also be used in cooking to add flavor and medicinal benefits.
- **Dosage**: The typical dosage for garlic supplements is 600–1,200 mg of standardized garlic extract per day. For fresh garlic, 1–2 cloves per day is recommended, either raw or lightly cooked.

Ginger (*Zingiber officinale*)

Ginger is not only known for its anti-inflammatory and digestive benefits, but also for its powerful antiviral and antibacterial effects. **Gingerol**, the active compound in ginger, has been found to inhibit the replication of viruses and bacteria in the body. Ginger is effective against respiratory infections, gastrointestinal infections, and even infections caused by drug-resistant bacteria. It also helps to stimulate the immune system and promote overall health, making it an excellent herb for combating both acute and chronic infections.

- **How to Use**: Fresh ginger can be used in teas, smoothies, or added to meals. It is also available in dried, powdered, or capsule form.
- **Dosage**: For therapeutic use, 1–2 grams of fresh ginger root or 500–1,000 mg of ginger extract can be taken daily.

Oregano (*Origanum vulgare*)

Oregano is well-known for its potent antibacterial, antiviral, and antifungal properties. The essential oil of oregano contains **carvacrol** and **thymol**, two powerful compounds that have been shown to inhibit the growth of harmful microorganisms, including **Staphylococcus aureus** and **Escherichia coli** (E. coli). Oregano has also demonstrated antiviral activity against a variety of viruses, including the flu and common cold. In addition to its antimicrobial effects, oregano supports digestive health and acts as a natural immune booster.

- **How to Use**: Oregano can be consumed fresh, dried, or in capsule or tincture form. Oregano oil is also used topically for treating skin infections.

- **Dosage:** For oregano oil, 200–500 mg of oregano oil extract can be taken 1–3 times per day. For fresh or dried oregano, 1–2 teaspoons can be added to meals or brewed as tea.

Andrographis (*Andrographis paniculata*)

Andrographis is a potent herb used in traditional medicine for its antiviral and antibacterial properties. It contains **andrographolide**, a compound known for its ability to inhibit the replication of both viruses and bacteria. Andrographis has been shown to be effective in treating upper respiratory infections, such as the common cold, flu, and even more severe conditions like **COVID-19**. In addition to its antimicrobial activity, Andrographis also boosts immune function, reduces inflammation, and supports overall wellness.

- **How to Use:** Andrographis is most commonly taken in capsule or tablet form, although it is also available as a tincture or extract.
- **Dosage:** The recommended dosage is typically 400–600 mg of andrographis extract per day, taken in divided doses.

Elderberry (*Sambucus nigra*)

Elderberry is widely known for its ability to fight viral infections, especially those caused by influenza. The active compounds in elderberry, such as **anthocyanins** and **flavonoids**, have been shown to prevent viruses from attaching to host cells, reducing the severity and duration of illnesses like the flu and colds. Elderberry also possesses antibacterial properties and supports the immune system, making it an excellent herb for both prevention and treatment of infections.

- **How to Use:** Elderberry can be taken as a syrup, extract, or in capsule form. It is also available as dried berries, which can be brewed into tea.
- **Dosage:** Elderberry syrup or extract is typically taken in doses of 1–2 teaspoons (5–10 mL) up to 3–4 times daily for acute infections. For prevention, a daily dose of 1 teaspoon is effective.

Lemon Balm (*Melissa officinalis*)

Lemon balm is a gentle yet effective herb that offers antiviral, antibacterial, and soothing properties. The active compound **rosmarinic acid** in lemon balm has been shown to fight viruses, particularly **herpes simplex virus (HSV)** and **human coronavirus**. It is also effective for reducing anxiety and promoting relaxation, making it an excellent herb for stress-related immune suppression. Lemon balm helps protect the body against a wide range of infections while calming the nervous system.

- **How to Use:** Lemon balm can be consumed as a tea, tincture, or in capsule form. It is also commonly used as a topical remedy for cold sores.
- **Dosage:** For therapeutic use, 1–2 teaspoons of dried lemon balm leaves can be steeped in hot water to make tea. Lemon balm extract is typically taken in doses of 300–600 mg per day.

Cat's Claw (*Uncaria tomentosa*)

Cat's Claw is a powerful herb traditionally used to treat viral infections and strengthen the immune system. Its active compounds, including **pentacyclic oxindole alkaloids (POAs)**, exhibit strong antiviral and antibacterial properties, making it effective in combating infections such as the common cold, flu, and even

HIV. Cat's Claw also supports immune modulation, enhancing the body's natural defenses without overstimulating the immune system.

- **How to Use**: Cat's Claw is typically consumed as a capsule, tablet, or tincture. It can also be brewed as a tea.
- **Dosage**: The typical dosage of Cat's Claw extract is 250–500 mg taken 1–2 times daily.

Tea Tree Oil (*Melaleuca alternifolia*)

Tea tree oil is a powerful antibacterial, antiviral, and antifungal essential oil known for its ability to combat a wide range of infections. It is most commonly used topically to treat skin infections, acne, fungal infections like athlete's foot, and even respiratory infections when inhaled. Tea tree oil's antimicrobial properties make it an excellent addition to your natural medicine cabinet, both for prevention and treatment of various infections.

- **How to Use**: Tea tree oil should always be diluted with a carrier oil before applying to the skin. It can also be used in steam inhalation or added to cleaning products.
- **Dosage**: For topical use, dilute 1–2 drops of tea tree oil with 1 teaspoon of carrier oil and apply to the affected area 2–3 times daily. For respiratory infections, add 5–10 drops to a diffuser or steam inhalation.

Bone and Joint Health Herbs

Our bones and joints are the foundation of our body's structure, enabling movement, flexibility, and support. However, as we age, wear and tear, injuries, and inflammatory conditions like arthritis can take a toll on bone and joint health. While conventional treatments are often used to manage joint pain and stiffness, nature offers a range of herbs that support bone density, strengthen cartilage, reduce inflammation, and promote overall joint health.

Herbs have been used for centuries to enhance mobility and prevent or alleviate the discomfort associated with bone and joint issues. Whether you're dealing with osteoarthritis, rheumatoid arthritis, or simply want to maintain strong bones and flexible joints as you age, incorporating these herbal remedies into your routine can help protect and rejuvenate your skeletal system.

Turmeric (*Curcuma longa*)

Turmeric, a golden-yellow root often used in cooking, is renowned for its anti-inflammatory and antioxidant properties. The active compound in turmeric, **curcumin**, has been extensively studied for its ability to reduce inflammation and pain in the joints, particularly in conditions like osteoarthritis and rheumatoid arthritis. Curcumin helps to inhibit the enzymes and cytokines that trigger inflammation, promoting joint mobility and reducing stiffness. Additionally, turmeric supports bone health by enhancing the activity of osteoblasts, the cells responsible for bone formation.

- **How to Use:** Turmeric can be taken as a spice in food, in smoothies, or in capsule and tincture form. It is often combined with black pepper to enhance absorption.
- **Dosage:** A typical dosage of standardized curcumin extract is 500–1,000 mg per day. For culinary use, 1–2 teaspoons of turmeric powder per day can be beneficial.

Boswellia (*Boswellia serrata*)

Boswellia, also known as **Indian frankincense**, is a potent herb commonly used in Ayurvedic medicine to treat joint pain and inflammation. Boswellia contains **boswellic acids**, which have been shown to reduce the production of pro-inflammatory enzymes and improve blood flow to the joints. Studies have found that Boswellia is effective in managing symptoms of osteoarthritis, rheumatoid arthritis, and other inflammatory joint conditions. It also promotes the regeneration of cartilage, which is vital for long-term joint health.

- **How to Use:** Boswellia is typically consumed in capsule or tablet form, although it is also available as a tincture or extract.
- **Dosage:** The recommended dosage of Boswellia extract is 300–500 mg, taken 2–3 times daily.

Devil's Claw (*Harpagophytum procumbens*)

Devil's Claw is an herb native to Southern Africa and has been used for centuries to treat pain and inflammation. The active compounds in Devil's Claw, particularly **harpagoside**, have demonstrated strong anti-inflammatory and analgesic properties. Devil's Claw has been found to be effective in reducing the pain and stiffness associated with osteoarthritis and rheumatoid arthritis, as well as other inflammatory conditions affecting the bones and joints.

- **How to Use:** Devil's Claw is most commonly taken in capsule, tablet, or tincture form, and it can also be used as a topical cream.
- **Dosage:** The typical dosage is 500–1,000 mg of standardized extract, taken 2–3 times daily.

Ginger (*Zingiber officinale*)

Ginger is another herb widely recognized for its anti-inflammatory properties, especially in relation to joint health. The active compounds in ginger, such as **gingerol**, have been shown to reduce inflammation and pain in the joints. Studies suggest that ginger may help to reduce symptoms of osteoarthritis and other inflammatory conditions by inhibiting the release of inflammatory substances like prostaglandins. Ginger also promotes blood circulation, which can enhance joint flexibility and mobility.

- **How to Use:** Ginger can be consumed fresh, dried, or in capsule form. It is commonly used in teas, smoothies, and meals.
- **Dosage:** For therapeutic use, 1–2 grams of fresh ginger root or 500–1,000 mg of ginger extract per day is recommended.

Alfalfa (*Medicago sativa*)

Alfalfa is a nutrient-dense herb that is rich in vitamins and minerals, including calcium, magnesium, and potassium—all of which are vital for bone health. Alfalfa is particularly beneficial in maintaining bone density and preventing bone loss, making it a valuable herb for those at risk of osteoporosis. In addition to its bone-strengthening properties, Alfalfa helps support joint health by reducing inflammation and improving mobility.

- **How to Use:** Alfalfa can be consumed as a tea, powder, or in capsule form. Alfalfa sprouts can also be added to salads and sandwiches for a fresh, nutritious boost.
- **Dosage:** The typical dosage is 500–1,000 mg of Alfalfa extract, taken 1–2 times daily.

Nettles (*Urtica dioica*)

Nettle, often referred to as **stinging nettle**, is a powerhouse herb that has been used for centuries to support joint and bone health. Nettle is rich in **silica** and **calcium**, two minerals that are essential for maintaining strong, healthy bones. It is also an anti-inflammatory herb that helps reduce joint pain, stiffness, and swelling, particularly in conditions like osteoarthritis and rheumatoid arthritis. Nettle also supports the kidneys and detoxifies the body, further promoting joint health by eliminating toxins that can exacerbate inflammation.

- **How to Use:** Nettle can be consumed as a tea, tincture, or in capsule form. Fresh nettles can also be added to soups or stews, but should be cooked to neutralize the sting.
- **Dosage:** For joint health, 1–2 teaspoons of dried nettle leaves can be brewed into tea 1–2 times per day. Alternatively, 300–600 mg of nettle extract can be taken daily.

White Willow Bark (*Salix alba*)

White Willow Bark has been used for centuries as a natural remedy for pain and inflammation. It contains **salicin**, a compound that is chemically similar to aspirin, which helps reduce pain, swelling, and inflammation in the joints. White Willow Bark is particularly effective in treating conditions like osteoarthritis and rheumatoid arthritis, as it targets pain at the root cause by reducing inflammation in the joints. It also promotes flexibility and mobility by soothing the tissues around the joints.

- **How to Use:** White Willow Bark can be taken as a tea, tincture, or in capsule form.
- **Dosage:** A typical dosage is 60–120 mg of salicin per day, taken in divided doses.

Horsetail (*Equisetum arvense*)

Horsetail is a herb rich in **silica**, a mineral that plays a crucial role in the formation and strength of bones, cartilage, and connective tissues. It is often used to help prevent bone loss and promote the healing of fractures. Horsetail also has anti-inflammatory properties that help to reduce joint pain and swelling. Its ability to improve the strength and flexibility of connective tissues makes it an excellent choice for joint and bone health.

- **How to Use:** Horsetail can be consumed as a tea, capsule, or tincture.
- **Dosage:** For general joint and bone support, 1–2 teaspoons of dried horsetail can be brewed into tea, or 300–500 mg of horsetail extract can be taken 1–2 times per day.

MSM (Methylsulfonylmethane)

While not an herb per se, **MSM** is a naturally occurring sulfur compound that is often included in herbal formulas to support joint health. MSM is known to reduce inflammation, alleviate pain, and promote the repair of damaged tissues, making it particularly beneficial for conditions like osteoarthritis and tendonitis. MSM also improves collagen production, which is essential for maintaining healthy cartilage, ligaments, and joints.

- **How to Use:** MSM is commonly available in powder, capsule, or tablet form.
- **Dosage:** A typical dosage is 1,000–3,000 mg of MSM per day, taken in divided doses.

Kidney and Urinary Health Herbs

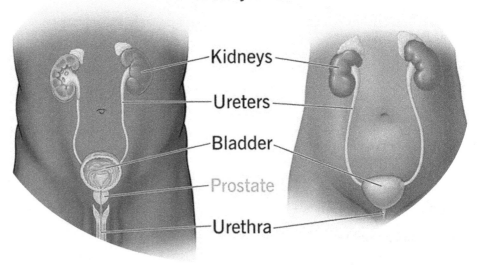

The kidneys and urinary system play a vital role in filtering waste, maintaining fluid and electrolyte balance, and supporting overall detoxification. Keeping these organs healthy is essential for the body's well-being. However, factors like poor diet, dehydration, infections, and toxins can put strain on the kidneys and urinary tract, leading to discomfort and a variety of health issues.

Herbs have long been used as natural remedies to support kidney and urinary health, offering gentle yet effective ways to detoxify, reduce inflammation, and support proper function. From cleansing the kidneys to soothing urinary tract irritation, certain herbs can provide essential benefits for maintaining a healthy urinary system.

Dandelion Root (*Taraxacum officinale*)

Dandelion, often considered a pesky weed, is a powerful herb with numerous health benefits. The root of the dandelion plant acts as a natural diuretic, stimulating the kidneys to expel excess fluid and waste without depleting vital electrolytes. In addition to its diuretic effects, dandelion root helps reduce inflammation in the kidneys and urinary tract, while promoting bile production, which aids in detoxification. This herb is particularly helpful for individuals with kidney stones, urinary tract infections (UTIs), or those looking to support general kidney health.

- **How to Use:** Dandelion root can be consumed as a tea, tincture, or in capsule form.
- **Dosage:** To support kidney and urinary health, 1–2 teaspoons of dried dandelion root can be brewed into tea 2–3 times per day, or 500–1,000 mg of dandelion root extract can be taken in capsule form.

Nettle Leaf (*Urtica dioica*)

Nettle leaf is an incredibly versatile herb that supports various aspects of kidney and urinary health. Known for its natural diuretic properties, nettle leaf helps flush toxins from the body while promoting the healthy function of the kidneys and bladder. It is especially beneficial for individuals dealing with urinary retention, kidney stones, or urinary tract infections. Nettle is also rich in vitamins and minerals, including iron, calcium, and magnesium, which nourish the kidneys and improve overall kidney function. Additionally, nettle leaf helps reduce inflammation in the urinary tract, soothing irritation and discomfort.

- **How to Use:** Nettle leaf can be consumed as a tea, tincture, or in capsule form. Fresh nettle leaves can also be added to soups and smoothies.
- **Dosage:** For urinary health, 1–2 teaspoons of dried nettle leaves can be brewed into tea 2–3 times per day, or 300–600 mg of nettle extract can be taken in capsule form daily.

Corn Silk (*Zea mays*)

Corn silk, the long threads that grow on the ears of corn, has been traditionally used to promote urinary health. This herb is especially beneficial for soothing urinary tract irritation, reducing inflammation, and supporting the smooth flow of urine. Corn silk acts as a gentle diuretic, helping to flush out waste from the kidneys while promoting healthy urine production. It is commonly used to relieve symptoms of urinary tract infections (UTIs), kidney stones, and benign prostate enlargement.

- **How to Use:** Corn silk can be consumed as a tea, tincture, or in capsule form.
- **Dosage:** To support urinary health, 1–2 teaspoons of dried corn silk can be brewed into tea 2–3 times per day, or 300–500 mg of corn silk extract can be taken in capsule form.

Cranberry (*Vaccinium macrocarpon*)

Cranberry is widely known for its ability to prevent and treat urinary tract infections (UTIs). The ac' compounds in cranberries, particularly **proanthocyanidins**, prevent harmful bacteria from adhering tc walls of the urinary tract, reducing the risk of infection. Cranberries are also rich in antioxidants, whic' reduce inflammation and protect the kidneys and urinary tract from oxidative damage. While cranber is commonly consumed for urinary health, cranberry supplements offer a more concentrated and effective dose.

- **How to Use:** Cranberry can be consumed as juice, in capsule form, or as a concentrated extract.
- **Dosage:** For UTI prevention, 400–500 mg of cranberry extract can be taken daily in capsule form. If using fresh cranberry juice, 1 cup per day is typically recommended.

Marshmallow Root (*Althaea officinalis*)

Marshmallow root is a soothing herb that is often used to relieve irritation and inflammation in the urinary tract. It contains **mucilage**, a gelatinous substance that forms a protective layer over the mucous membranes, reducing discomfort and promoting healing in the bladder and kidneys. Marshmallow root is especially useful for individuals experiencing frequent urination, bladder infections, or kidney irritation. Its mild diuretic effect helps cleanse the kidneys while keeping the urinary tract well-hydrated.

- **How to Use:** Marshmallow root can be taken as a tea, tincture, or in capsule form.
- **Dosage:** To soothe the urinary system, 1–2 teaspoons of dried marshmallow root can be brewed into tea 2–3 times daily, or 500–1,000 mg of marshmallow root extract can be taken in capsule form.

Parsley (*Petroselinum crispum*)

Parsley is not only a popular culinary herb but also a powerful diuretic that promotes kidney health and helps eliminate toxins from the body. It stimulates urine production, which helps flush waste and excess fluids from the kidneys and urinary tract. Parsley also contains **flavonoids** and **vitamin C**, which act as antioxidants, protecting the kidneys from oxidative stress. This herb is often used as a natural remedy for kidney stones, urinary tract infections, and general detoxification.

- **How to Use:** Parsley can be consumed fresh in salads or smoothies, or as a tea. It is also available in capsule or tincture form.
- **Dosage:** For kidney health, 1–2 teaspoons of dried parsley leaves can be brewed into tea 1–2 times per day, or 500 mg of parsley extract can be taken in capsule form daily.

Hydrangea Root (*Hydrangea arborescens*)

Hydrangea root has been traditionally used to support kidney health and prevent kidney stones. It contains **saponins** and **flavonoids**, which help reduce inflammation, promote detoxification, and support proper urinary flow. Hydrangea root is also believed to help break down and prevent the formation of kidney stones, making it a valuable herb for individuals prone to these painful deposits. Additionally, hydrangea is known to promote overall kidney function by helping to balance electrolytes and encourage the elimination of waste.

- **How to Use:** Hydrangea root can be consumed in capsule, tincture, or tea form.
- **Dosage:** The recommended dosage is typically 500–1,000 mg of hydrangea extract, taken 2–3 times daily.

Uva Ursi (*Arctostaphylos uva-ursi*)

Uva Ursi, also known as **bearberry**, is a powerful herb used for treating urinary tract infections (UTIs) and promoting urinary tract health. It contains **arbutin**, a compound that has antimicrobial and astringent properties, helping to cleanse the urinary tract by inhibiting bacterial growth. Uva Ursi is particularly effective for treating bladder infections, as it helps to reduce inflammation and relieve symptoms like burning or frequent urination.

- **How to Use**: Uva Ursi is typically consumed in capsule, tincture, or tea form.
- **Dosage**: For UTIs, 400–800 mg of Uva Ursi extract can be taken daily, or 1–2 teaspoons of dried leaves can be brewed into tea 2–3 times per day.

Ginger (*Zingiber officinale*)

Ginger, well-known for its anti-inflammatory and digestive benefits, also supports kidney and urinary health by promoting detoxification and reducing inflammation. Its active compound, **gingerol**, has been shown to improve kidney function and protect against oxidative stress. Ginger is especially helpful for individuals with urinary tract infections, kidney stones, and general kidney discomfort, as it aids in the natural flushing of toxins and supports overall kidney health.

- **How to Use**: Ginger can be consumed fresh, dried, or in capsule form. It is also commonly used in teas, smoothies, and meals.
- **Dosage**: For kidney and urinary health, 1–2 grams of fresh ginger root or 500–1,000 mg of ginger extract per day is recommended.

Stress and Anxiety Relief Herbs

In today's fast-paced world, stress and anxiety have become all too common, affecting millions of people worldwide. Whether caused by work pressures, personal challenges, or the demands of modern life, chronic stress can have a profound impact on both physical and mental health. Fortunately, nature offers a range of herbs that can help soothe the mind, calm the nerves, and promote a sense of balance and well-being.

Herbal remedies for stress and anxiety have been used for centuries, with many traditional cultures relying on plants for their calming, mood-lifting, and anxiolytic (anxiety-reducing) properties. From promoting relaxation to improving sleep quality, the right herbs can provide effective, natural support for managing the stresses of daily life.

Ashwagandha (*Withania somnifera*)

Ashwagandha is a highly revered herb in Ayurvedic medicine, known for its ability to combat stress and improve resilience to daily pressures. As an **adaptogen**, Ashwagandha helps the body adapt to stress by regulating the adrenal glands and balancing cortisol levels—the hormone responsible for the body's stress response. Regular use of Ashwagandha can promote a calm, grounded sense of well-being, enhance mood, and support overall mental clarity. Studies have shown that Ashwagandha can effectively reduce symptoms of anxiety, depression, and chronic stress, making it a powerful tool in managing emotional health.

- **How to Use:** Ashwagandha is typically available in capsule, powder, or liquid extract form. It can also be added to smoothies or teas.

- **Dosage:** A typical dose of Ashwagandha extract is 300–500 mg per day, taken 1–2 times daily. For powder form, 1–2 teaspoons per day is commonly recommended.

Lavender (*Lavandula angustifolia*)

Lavender is one of the most widely used herbs for relaxation, offering both calming and anti-anxiety properties. Its **linalool** and **linalyl acetate** compounds have been shown to reduce the physical symptoms of stress, including muscle tension and heart palpitations, while also promoting mental relaxation. Lavender is often used to alleviate anxiety, insomnia, and restlessness. Its soothing scent is frequently used in aromatherapy, but lavender can also be consumed in tea or as an essential oil for a more direct effect.

- **How to Use:** Lavender can be used as a tea, essential oil (for diffusing or topical application), or in capsule form. Lavender tea is especially calming before bedtime.

- **Dosage:** For anxiety relief, 1–2 capsules of lavender extract (80 mg) or 1–2 cups of lavender tea per day are effective. For essential oil use, 4-6 drops in a diffuser or a few drops diluted in carrier oil for topical use can be beneficial.

Chamomile (*Matricaria recutita*)

Chamomile has long been known for its gentle sedative effects, making it one of the most popular herbs for relaxation and stress relief. It contains **apigenin**, a flavonoid that binds to specific receptors in the brain, helping to calm the nervous system and reduce feelings of anxiety. Chamomile is particularly helpful for those struggling with insomnia, nervous tension, or irritability, as it promotes a deep sense of calm and mental clarity.

- **How to Use:** Chamomile is commonly consumed as a tea, but it is also available in tincture and capsule forms.

- **Dosage:** Drinking 1–2 cups of chamomile tea per day is an effective way to reduce anxiety. Alternatively, 300–400 mg of chamomile extract can be taken in capsule form.

Passionflower (*Passiflora incarnata*)

Passionflower is a calming herb that has been traditionally used to treat anxiety, stress, and insomnia. It contains **harmine** and **harmaline**, compounds that help increase the availability of **gamma-aminobutyric acid** (GABA), a neurotransmitter that promotes relaxation and reduces brain activity associated with stress and anxiety. Passionflower is particularly effective for people who experience racing thoughts, irritability, or difficulty unwinding after a stressful day.

- **How to Use:** Passionflower is most commonly taken in tincture, tea, or capsule form. It can also be used as an extract.

- **Dosage**: For general stress and anxiety relief, 200–400 mg of Passionflower extract, or 1–2 cups of Passionflower tea per day, is recommended.

Lemon Balm (*Melissa officinalis*)

Lemon balm, a member of the mint family, is known for its mood-boosting and anxiety-reducing properties. It contains **rosmarinic acid**, which helps reduce the effects of stress by calming the nervous system and reducing the intensity of physical symptoms such as heart palpitations and restlessness. Lemon balm is often used to reduce symptoms of anxiety, promote mental clarity, and improve sleep quality.

- **How to Use**: Lemon balm is most commonly consumed as a tea, but it is also available in capsule and tincture forms.
- **Dosage**: 1–2 cups of lemon balm tea, or 300–500 mg of lemon balm extract per day, can help alleviate anxiety and promote relaxation.

Rhodiola (*Rhodiola rosea*)

Rhodiola is another adaptogenic herb that enhances the body's ability to manage stress and improve mental performance under pressure. Known for its ability to combat both physical and mental fatigue, Rhodiola helps regulate the body's stress response by balancing cortisol levels and promoting the production of mood-boosting neurotransmitters like serotonin and dopamine. Rhodiola can help increase energy, focus, and resilience, while also reducing anxiety and improving overall emotional well-being.

- **How to Use**: Rhodiola is typically taken in capsule, powder, or liquid extract form.
- **Dosage**: A standard dosage for Rhodiola is 200–400 mg of extract per day, taken in the morning or early afternoon.

Valerian Root (*Valeriana officinalis*)

Valerian root is a well-known herb for promoting relaxation and improving sleep quality. It works by increasing the levels of **GABA** in the brain, which has a calming effect on the nervous system. Valerian root is particularly useful for those who experience stress-induced insomnia or heightened anxiety at night. It has mild sedative effects that can help reduce nervous tension and promote restful sleep without the risk of dependency commonly associated with pharmaceutical sleep aids.

- **How to Use**: Valerian root can be taken as a tea, capsule, or tincture.
- **Dosage**: For anxiety or sleep support, 300–600 mg of valerian root extract can be taken 30 minutes before bedtime. Alternatively, 1–2 cups of valerian root tea can be consumed in the evening.

Holy Basil (*Ocimum sanctum* or *Ocimum tenuiflorum*)

Holy Basil, also known as **Tulsi**, is a sacred herb in Ayurvedic medicine that helps the body adapt to stress and enhance emotional resilience. Holy Basil is a potent adaptogen that helps balance cortisol levels, reduce the effects of stress, and promote mental clarity. It has anti-inflammatory properties that support overall well-being and can enhance the body's ability to recover from stress-related physical ailments.

- **How to Use**: Holy Basil is available in tea, tincture, capsule, or powder form.

- **Dosage**: To manage stress, 300–600 mg of Holy Basil extract can be taken daily, or 1–2 cups of Holy Basil tea can be consumed.

Magnolia Bark (*Magnolia officinalis*)

Magnolia bark has been traditionally used in Chinese medicine to alleviate stress and anxiety. It contains **honokiol** and **magnolol**, compounds that help reduce cortisol levels and promote relaxation. Magnolia bark is effective in calming the mind, alleviating stress, and reducing symptoms of anxiety, especially when used as part of an overall stress management routine.

- **How to Use**: Magnolia bark is available in capsule, tincture, or powdered form.
- **Dosage**: A typical dosage is 200–400 mg of Magnolia bark extract per day, taken in divided doses.

Hair and Scalp Health Herbs

The health of your hair and scalp is a reflection of your overall well-being. From maintaining a healthy scalp environment to nourishing hair follicles, proper care is essential for promoting hair growth, reducing hair loss, and improving the overall appearance of your hair. While various factors such as genetics, nutrition, stress, and environmental conditions can impact hair health, nature offers a wealth of herbs that can support and enhance the health of both your hair and scalp.

Herbal remedies for hair and scalp health have been used for centuries in traditional medicine, valued for their ability to nourish, strengthen, and rejuvenate hair. Whether you're dealing with dryness, dandruff, hair thinning, or an irritated scalp, these herbs can provide effective, natural solutions to restore balance and promote healthy hair growth.

Rosemary (*Rosmarinus officinalis*)

Rosemary is one of the most well-known herbs for stimulating hair growth and improving scalp health. Rich in antioxidants and essential nutrients, **rosemary** helps increase circulation to the scalp, which in turn promotes healthy hair follicles and encourages hair growth. It also has anti-inflammatory and antimicrobial properties that can help combat dandruff, itching, and scalp irritation. Rosemary is often used in hair oils, shampoos, and as a topical infusion to promote thicker, shinier hair.

- **How to Use**: Rosemary can be applied directly to the scalp in the form of essential oil diluted in a carrier oil, used as a rinse, or added to hair care products.
- **Dosage**: To use rosemary oil, dilute 3-5 drops of essential rosemary oil in 1 tablespoon of carrier oil (like coconut or jojoba oil) and massage into the scalp for 5–10 minutes, leaving it on for at least 30 minutes before washing out. Alternatively, use rosemary-infused water as a final rinse after shampooing.

Nettle (*Urtica dioica*)

Nettle is a powerhouse herb for hair health, thanks to its rich content of vitamins, minerals, and fatty acids that nourish the scalp and promote strong hair. Nettle is especially effective in treating scalp conditions like dandruff, itching, and irritation due to its **anti-inflammatory** properties. It also contains high levels of **silica** and **sulfur**, which help strengthen hair, reduce hair loss, and improve hair texture. Nettle is also believed to help balance hormones, which can be especially beneficial for people experiencing hair loss due to hormonal imbalances.

- **How to Use**: Nettle is commonly used in the form of tea, tinctures, or applied topically in hair rinses.
- **Dosage**: For general hair and scalp health, drink 1–2 cups of nettle tea per day, or use nettle extract (300–600 mg) in capsule form. For topical application, prepare a nettle infusion and use it as a hair rinse after shampooing.

Peppermint (*Mentha piperita*)

Peppermint is a stimulating herb known for its invigorating effects on the scalp. The menthol in peppermint oil helps increase blood flow to the scalp, which promotes hair growth and strengthens hair follicles. It also has a cooling and soothing effect on the scalp, making it effective for alleviating itching and reducing dandruff. The antimicrobial properties of peppermint oil help keep the scalp clean and free from bacteria, which is essential for maintaining a healthy hair growth environment.

- **How to Use**: Peppermint oil can be used in scalp massages, hair masks, or added to your regular shampoo.
- **Dosage**: To use peppermint oil, dilute 3-5 drops of essential peppermint oil in a carrier oil and massage it into the scalp. Leave it for about 15–20 minutes before rinsing. You can also add 2-3 drops to your shampoo or conditioner for an invigorating effect.

Saw Palmetto (*Serenoa repens*)

Saw Palmetto is a well-known herb for promoting hair growth and reducing hair thinning, especially in cases of **androgenetic alopecia** (male or female pattern baldness). It works by inhibiting the enzyme **5-alpha reductase**, which converts testosterone into **dihydrotestosterone** (DHT), a hormone responsible for hair loss. By blocking DHT production, Saw Palmetto can help prevent hair follicles from shrinking, promoting healthier, thicker hair growth. It is also thought to support scalp health by reducing inflammation and promoting circulation.

- **How to Use**: Saw Palmetto is commonly used as a supplement in capsule or liquid extract form.
- **Dosage**: A typical dose is 320 mg of Saw Palmetto extract per day, which can be divided into two doses.

Horsetail (*Equisetum arvense*)

Horsetail is a mineral-rich herb that has long been used to promote healthy hair, nails, and skin. It is particularly high in **silica**, an essential mineral that helps strengthen hair strands and promote elasticity. Silica also supports healthy collagen production, which is important for the strength and structure of hair follicles.

Horsetail is effective in treating hair thinning and loss, and can help improve overall hair texture and shine by nourishing the scalp and hair follicles.

- **How to Use:** Horsetail can be taken as a tea, tincture, or in capsule form.
- **Dosage:** To promote hair health, take 300–500 mg of horsetail extract per day, or drink 1–2 cups of horsetail tea daily. For topical use, horsetail-infused oil can be massaged into the scalp.

Aloe Vera (*Aloe barbadensis miller*)

Aloe vera is a soothing herb that is commonly used to treat scalp conditions such as dryness, flakiness, and dandruff. It contains **enzymes** that help exfoliate the scalp, promoting healthier hair growth by removing dead skin cells. Aloe vera also has **anti-inflammatory** properties that can soothe an irritated scalp and reduce inflammation caused by conditions like seborrheic dermatitis or psoriasis. Its high moisture content helps to hydrate the scalp and keep hair strands nourished and shiny.

- **How to Use:** Aloe vera gel can be applied directly to the scalp or mixed with oils for a hydrating hair mask.
- **Dosage:** To use aloe vera on the scalp, apply fresh aloe vera gel directly to the scalp, massaging it in for 10–15 minutes. Leave it on for at least 30 minutes before washing it out.

Burdock Root (*Arctium lappa*)

Burdock root has been used for centuries to promote hair growth and improve scalp health. Rich in essential fatty acids, **inulin**, and **antioxidants**, it helps nourish hair follicles and improve circulation to the scalp. Burdock root is particularly useful for treating scalp conditions such as dandruff, itching, and dryness, as it helps detoxify the scalp and remove toxins. It is also known to strengthen hair and improve its overall texture.

- **How to Use:** Burdock root is commonly consumed in tea, tincture, or capsule form, and can also be used as a topical infusion for hair rinses.
- **Dosage:** For internal use, drink 1–2 cups of burdock root tea daily, or take 500–1,000 mg of burdock root extract in capsule form. For topical use, prepare a burdock root infusion and apply it to the scalp as a rinse after shampooing.

Ginseng (*Panax ginseng*)

Ginseng is a well-known herb for its ability to boost energy and vitality, but it also offers significant benefits for hair health. It improves blood circulation to the scalp, which helps deliver essential nutrients to hair follicles, stimulating hair growth. Ginseng also contains **ginsenosides**, compounds that help rejuvenate the scalp, reduce hair loss, and promote the overall health of hair follicles. It can be especially helpful for individuals with thinning hair or those recovering from stress-related hair loss.

- **How to Use:** Ginseng can be consumed as a supplement, or used in topical treatments such as shampoos or hair tonics.
- **Dosage:** The typical dose of ginseng extract is 200–400 mg per day, which can be divided into two doses. For topical application, ginseng-infused oil or extract can be massaged into the scalp.

Jojoba Oil (*Simmondsia chinensis*)

Jojoba oil is a versatile and nourishing oil that mimics the natural oils produced by the scalp, making it ideal for maintaining scalp health and hydration. It is rich in **vitamins E and B**, as well as **minerals** like copper and zinc, which help strengthen hair and promote healthy growth. Jojoba oil helps balance sebum production, preventing both dry scalp and excess oil, and it can also help soothe scalp irritation and dandruff.

- **How to Use:** Jojoba oil can be massaged into the scalp or added to hair care products like shampoos and conditioners.
- **Dosage:** For scalp treatment, massage a small amount of jojoba oil (1-2 teaspoons) into the scalp and leave it on for 30 minutes before washing. It can also be used as a leave-in treatment for dry or frizzy hair.

Circulatory Health Herbs

The circulatory system is responsible for transporting blood, oxygen, and nutrients throughout the body. Maintaining a healthy circulatory system is essential for overall well-being, as it supports every organ and tissue. Poor circulation, if left unaddressed, can lead to a range of health issues, including fatigue, cold extremities, high blood pressure, varicose veins, and an increased risk of cardiovascular diseases.

Herbal remedies have long been used to support and improve circulation, strengthen the heart, and promote vascular health. Many herbs are packed with antioxidants, flavonoids, and other bioactive compounds that can enhance blood flow, reduce inflammation, and help keep arteries and veins flexible and strong.

Hawthorn (*Crataegus spp.*)

Hawthorn is a time-tested herb for promoting heart health and improving circulation. Rich in antioxidants, including flavonoids like **quercetin** and **proanthocyanidins**, hawthorn has been shown to help dilate blood vessels, improve blood flow, and reduce blood pressure. It supports the heart by strengthening the heart muscles, improving cardiac output, and enhancing the efficiency of the circulatory system. Hawthorn is also used to support healthy cholesterol levels and reduce inflammation, making it an excellent choice for cardiovascular wellness.

- **How to Use:** Hawthorn can be taken as a tincture, capsule, tea, or extract.
- **Dosage:** A typical dose for hawthorn extract is 250–500 mg, taken 1–3 times per day. For tea, drink 1–2 cups daily.

Garlic (*Allium sativum*)

Garlic is widely known for its numerous health benefits, particularly for cardiovascular health. It contains **allicin**, a sulfur compound that has been shown to improve circulation by promoting the dilation of blood vessels and reducing the formation of blood clots. Garlic also helps lower **blood pressure**, regulate **cholesterol levels**, and reduce **arterial plaque**, thus supporting overall circulatory function. In addition to its circulatory benefits, garlic has powerful **anti-inflammatory** and **antioxidant** properties that help protect the vascular system from oxidative damage.

- **How to Use:** Garlic can be consumed raw, in food, as a supplement, or in tincture form.
- **Dosage:** For general circulatory health, 1–2 cloves of raw garlic per day are recommended. If using garlic supplements, a dose of 600–1,200 mg of standardized garlic extract per day is common.

Ginkgo Biloba (*Ginkgo biloba*)

Ginkgo biloba is one of the most well-known herbs for improving circulation and supporting cognitive health. It works by enhancing blood flow to the brain and extremities through its ability to **dilate blood vessels** and improve blood vessel flexibility. Ginkgo also promotes the health of the endothelial cells that line blood vessels, improving circulation and reducing the risk of blood clots. It has been found to be especially helpful for people with **peripheral vascular disease**, a condition characterized by reduced blood flow to the legs and arms.

- **How to Use:** Ginkgo is commonly available in capsules, tablets, or liquid extract form.
- **Dosage:** For circulatory health, a dose of 120–240 mg of standardized ginkgo extract per day is commonly used, taken in divided doses.

Ginger (*Zingiber officinale*)

Ginger is a well-loved herb with powerful circulatory benefits. It promotes healthy blood circulation by stimulating the **heart and blood vessels**, helping to maintain optimal blood flow throughout the body. Ginger also has natural **anti-inflammatory** and **antioxidant** properties that can reduce oxidative stress and prevent the buildup of plaque in the arteries. This makes it an excellent herb for cardiovascular support, as well as for improving circulation in cold extremities, such as hands and feet.

- **How to Use:** Ginger can be consumed fresh, as a powder, or as a supplement. It can also be brewed as a tea or used in cooking.
- **Dosage:** A typical dose of ginger extract ranges from 500 mg to 1,000 mg per day, or 1–2 teaspoons of fresh ginger root in tea daily.

Cayenne Pepper (*Capsicum annuum*)

Cayenne pepper, often known for its spicy heat, is also an excellent herb for improving circulation. It contains **capsaicin**, a compound that stimulates blood flow by promoting the dilation of blood vessels and improving the overall functioning of the circulatory system. Cayenne also has natural **anti-inflammatory** properties and is known to support heart health by helping to lower **blood pressure**, reduce **cholesterol levels**, and improve overall circulation to the extremities.

- **How to Use:** Cayenne can be used in cooking, as a supplement, or in tincture form.
- **Dosage:** As a supplement, a typical dose of cayenne extract is 30–120 mg per day. If using cayenne pepper in cooking, adding 1/4 to 1/2 teaspoon to your meals can provide circulatory benefits.

Bilberry (*Vaccinium myrtillus*)

Bilberry is rich in **anthocyanins**, powerful antioxidants that promote the health of blood vessels and improve circulation. By supporting the integrity of the vascular walls, bilberry helps to enhance blood flow and reduce the risk of vascular conditions such as varicose veins and hemorrhoids. Bilberry has also been shown to support the strength and flexibility of capillaries, which is essential for overall circulatory health and preventing conditions related to poor blood flow.

- **How to Use:** Bilberry is available as an extract, capsule, or in dried form to make tea.
- **Dosage:** The recommended dosage of bilberry extract is 80–160 mg, taken 1–2 times per day. For tea, 1–2 teaspoons of dried bilberry can be steeped in hot water.

Beetroot (*Beta vulgaris*)

Beetroot is a powerful food and herb known for its ability to improve blood circulation. It contains high levels of **nitrates**, which the body converts into **nitric oxide**, a molecule that relaxes and dilates blood vessels, improving blood flow. This process helps lower **blood pressure** and enhances overall cardiovascular function. Beetroot also supports healthy red blood cell production and increases oxygen transport throughout the body, contributing to better endurance and vitality.

- **How to Use:** Beetroot can be consumed raw, juiced, or as a supplement.
- **Dosage:** For circulatory health, 1/2 to 1 cup of fresh beetroot juice or beetroot powder (1–2 teaspoons) per day can be beneficial.

Turmeric (*Curcuma longa*)

Turmeric is a powerful herb widely recognized for its **anti-inflammatory** and **antioxidant** properties, both of which support cardiovascular health. The active compound in turmeric, **curcumin**, has been shown to improve blood circulation by reducing inflammation in the blood vessels, preventing the buildup of arterial plaque, and enhancing endothelial function. Turmeric also helps reduce **blood pressure** and may aid in lowering cholesterol levels, making it a valuable herb for overall circulatory health.

- **How to Use:** Turmeric can be consumed in food, as a supplement, or used as a powder to make a soothing tea or "golden milk."
- **Dosage:** A common dose of turmeric extract is 500–1,000 mg of standardized curcumin per day. To make a turmeric tea, mix 1 teaspoon of turmeric powder in warm water with honey and lemon.

Green Tea (*Camellia sinensis*)

Green tea is not only a refreshing beverage but also an excellent herb for supporting circulatory health. It is rich in **catechins**, particularly **epigallocatechin gallate** (EGCG), which have been shown to improve blood vessel health, reduce inflammation, and lower blood pressure. Green tea also helps maintain healthy cholesterol levels and supports the prevention of atherosclerosis (hardening of the arteries), making it a great herb for long-term heart and circulatory support.

- **How to Use:** Green tea is best consumed as a beverage, either hot or cold. It is also available as a supplement or extract.

- **Dosage:** To reap circulatory benefits, drink 2–3 cups of green tea per day, or take 300–500 mg of green tea extract as a supplement.

Mood & Cognitive Support Herbs

Mental clarity, emotional stability, and cognitive function are crucial elements of overall well-being. The demands of daily life—stress, aging, fatigue, and environmental factors—can take a toll on the brain and mood, leading to difficulties with focus, memory, concentration, and emotional balance. Fortunately, nature offers a variety of herbs that can support both cognitive function and emotional well-being, helping to maintain mental sharpness, enhance mood, and alleviate stress.

Herbs for mood and cognitive support have been used for centuries in traditional medicine to help uplift the spirit, enhance mental clarity, reduce anxiety, and support the nervous system. These herbs work in diverse ways—some improve blood flow to the brain, while others balance neurotransmitters or support the body's ability to cope with stress.

Rhodiola (*Rhodiola rosea*)

Rhodiola, often called "the golden root," is an adaptogenic herb known for its ability to help the body adapt to stress while boosting mental and physical performance. By increasing the production of serotonin, dopamine, and norepinephrine, Rhodiola helps regulate mood, improve cognitive function, and alleviate fatigue. It's particularly beneficial for individuals dealing with stress-related cognitive decline or emotional fatigue. Rhodiola is also known to enhance memory, focus, and mental resilience, making it an excellent herb for improving overall cognitive performance.

- **How to Use:** Rhodiola is commonly consumed as a capsule, tablet, tincture, or powder.
- **Dosage:** A typical dose is 200–400 mg of Rhodiola extract per day, taken in the morning or early afternoon. It is important not to take Rhodiola too late in the day, as it may interfere with sleep.

Ginkgo Biloba (*Ginkgo biloba*)

Ginkgo biloba is one of the oldest living tree species and has been used for centuries to support cognitive health and improve mental clarity. Ginkgo works by enhancing blood flow to the brain and increasing the delivery of oxygen and nutrients to brain cells, which helps improve memory, focus, and mental sharpness. It also has antioxidant properties, protecting brain cells from oxidative stress and supporting overall cognitive function. Ginkgo is often used by individuals looking to improve focus, combat age-related cognitive decline, and promote emotional well-being.

- **How to Use:** Ginkgo is most commonly available as a supplement (capsules, tablets, or liquid extracts) or as dried leaves for making tea.
- **Dosage:** The typical recommended dose is 120–240 mg of standardized Ginkgo biloba extract per day, divided into 1–2 doses.

Ashwagandha (*Withania somnifera*)

Ashwagandha is another powerful adaptogen known for its ability to support the nervous system and improve cognitive function. It works by regulating the body's stress response, lowering cortisol levels, and helping to balance the thyroid and adrenal glands. By stabilizing mood and reducing anxiety, Ashwagandha helps improve mental clarity, focus, and concentration. Additionally, studies have shown that Ashwagandha can improve memory, enhance learning capacity, and support overall cognitive health, especially in cases of stress-related cognitive decline.

- **How to Use:** Ashwagandha is available in capsules, powders, and tinctures, and can also be consumed as a tea.
- **Dosage:** A typical dose is 300–600 mg of Ashwagandha extract per day, often taken in two doses. For powdered Ashwagandha, 1–2 teaspoons per day is common.

Bacopa (*Bacopa monnieri*)

Bacopa, also known as **Brahmi**, has been used in Ayurvedic medicine for centuries to enhance cognitive function, memory, and learning ability. Bacopa supports brain health by increasing the synthesis of **acetylcholine**, a neurotransmitter involved in memory and learning processes. It also has **antioxidant** and **anti-inflammatory** effects, which help protect the brain from age-related cognitive decline and oxidative damage. Bacopa is particularly beneficial for improving mental clarity, concentration, and overall cognitive performance.

- **How to Use:** Bacopa is commonly found in capsule, tablet, or liquid extract form. It can also be brewed as a tea.
- **Dosage:** A typical dose of Bacopa extract is 300–450 mg per day, divided into 1–2 doses. Bacopa may take several weeks of consistent use to show noticeable cognitive benefits.

St. John's Wort (*Hypericum perforatum*)

St. John's Wort is a well-known herb used to support emotional well-being and balance mood. It is particularly effective for individuals dealing with mild to moderate depression, anxiety, and mood swings. St. John's Wort works by increasing the levels of serotonin, dopamine, and norepinephrine in the brain, helping to improve mood and reduce feelings of sadness and stress. It has been used for centuries to address symptoms of depression and anxiety, offering a natural alternative to pharmaceutical antidepressants.

- **How to Use:** St. John's Wort is commonly available in capsule, tablet, or tincture form.
- **Dosage:** A typical dosage of St. John's Wort extract ranges from 300–900 mg per day, often divided into two or three doses. It is important to consult with a healthcare provider before using St. John's Wort, especially if taking other medications, as it may interact with certain drugs.

Lemon Balm (*Melissa officinalis*)

Lemon balm is a calming herb that has been used for centuries to relieve stress, reduce anxiety, and improve mental clarity. It works by increasing the levels of **GABA** (gamma-aminobutyric acid) in the brain, a neurotransmitter that promotes relaxation and reduces the impact of stress. Lemon balm also has mild

antioxidant properties, which support brain health by protecting cells from oxidative damage. Its soothing effects can improve focus, alleviate nervous tension, and promote a balanced, clear mind.

- **How to Use:** Lemon balm is typically consumed as a tea, tincture, or in capsule form.
- **Dosage:** For anxiety and mood support, a dose of 300–500 mg of lemon balm extract per day is common. Alternatively, drink 1–2 cups of lemon balm tea daily for calming effects.

Gotu Kola (*Centella Asiatica*)

Gotu Kola is an herb that is widely used in traditional medicine to support brain function, mental clarity, and cognitive performance. It enhances memory, focus, and concentration by improving blood flow to the brain and supporting the integrity of the blood-brain barrier. Gotu Kola also has **neuroprotective** properties, helping to protect brain cells from age-related damage and oxidative stress. It is often used as a tonic to promote mental clarity and enhance overall cognitive function.

- **How to Use:** Gotu Kola is available in capsules, tablets, or as a liquid tincture. It can also be brewed as a tea.
- **Dosage:** A common dose of Gotu Kola is 300–500 mg of extract per day, or 1–2 teaspoons of dried herb brewed as a tea.

Turmeric (*Curcuma longa*)

Turmeric, known for its powerful anti-inflammatory and antioxidant properties, is also beneficial for brain health and mood regulation. The active compound in turmeric, **curcumin**, has been shown to enhance cognitive function, reduce the effects of stress, and improve overall brain health. Curcumin supports the production of **BDNF** (brain-derived neurotrophic factor), a protein that promotes the growth and maintenance of brain cells. It can also help reduce symptoms of anxiety and depression, making it a powerful herb for emotional well-being.

- **How to Use:** Turmeric can be consumed as a supplement, used in cooking, or brewed into a soothing tea.
- **Dosage:** For cognitive and mood support, a typical dose of **curcumin** extract is 500–1,000 mg per day. If using turmeric powder, 1–2 teaspoons per day is common.

Schisandra (*Schisandra chinensis*)

Schisandra is an adaptogenic herb that helps the body cope with stress and enhances mental clarity and focus. Known as the "five-flavor fruit" for its complex flavor profile, Schisandra promotes cognitive performance by increasing mental alertness and focus while reducing the impact of stress on the body. It also supports liver health, which is crucial for maintaining mental clarity and emotional stability. Schisandra helps to balance mood, increase energy, and improve overall cognitive function, making it a powerful herb for both mental and physical vitality.

- **How to Use:** Schisandra is commonly available as a supplement (capsules, tablets) or as a tincture.
- **Dosage:** A typical dose of Schisandra extract ranges from 500 mg to 1,000 mg per day, taken in divided doses.

Sexual Health & Libido Herbs

Sexual health and libido are integral components of overall well-being, playing an essential role in emotional and physical vitality, as well as intimate relationships. However, factors such as stress, hormonal imbalances, aging, lifestyle choices, and physical health can affect sexual drive and performance. Fortunately, many herbs offer natural solutions to support sexual health, enhance libido, and promote reproductive function.

Herbs for sexual health work in a variety of ways. Some increase blood circulation to the reproductive organs, while others balance hormones, reduce stress, or improve overall vitality. Many of these herbs have been used for centuries in traditional medicine to help boost energy, enhance libido, and address sexual dysfunction.

Maca (*Lepidium meyenii*)

Maca, often referred to as "Peruvian ginseng," is a root herb native to the Andes, widely celebrated for its ability to enhance sexual function and boost libido. Known for its adaptogenic properties, Maca helps balance hormones and improve energy levels, making it a great herb for those experiencing low sexual desire due to stress, fatigue, or hormonal imbalance. Maca has been shown to increase sexual desire, improve erectile function, and promote fertility in both men and women. It is particularly useful for boosting energy, mood, and overall vitality.

- **How to Use:** Maca is commonly available as a powder, capsule, or tincture. It can be added to smoothies, shakes, or teas.
- **Dosage:** A typical dose of Maca powder is 1.5–3 grams per day, while capsules usually contain 500–1,000 mg per dose.

Tribulus Terrestris (*Tribulus terrestris*)

Tribulus Terrestris is a powerful herb used to support libido, increase energy, and improve overall sexual performance. It is particularly popular among athletes and individuals experiencing low libido or sexual dysfunction. Tribulus works by increasing the production of **luteinizing hormone**, which in turn stimulates the production of testosterone, a key hormone responsible for sexual desire and function in both men and women. It has also been shown to improve erectile function and enhance sexual pleasure.

- **How to Use:** Tribulus is typically available in capsules, tablets, or tincture form.
- **Dosage:** The typical recommended dose of Tribulus Terrestris extract is 250–500 mg per day, taken in divided doses.

Horny Goat Weed (*Epimedium spp.*)

Horny Goat Weed, also known as **Epimedium**, is an herb that has been traditionally used in Chinese medicine to enhance libido, improve sexual performance, and increase energy. The active compound in Horny Goat Weed, **icariin**, is believed to improve blood flow to the genital area by inhibiting the enzyme that restricts nitric oxide production. This helps to enhance sexual function, improve erectile performance, and increase sexual desire. Horny Goat Weed is especially beneficial for individuals dealing with erectile dysfunction or reduced libido due to aging or hormonal changes.

- **How to Use:** Horny Goat Weed is available in capsules, tablets, or as a liquid extract.
- **Dosage:** A typical dose of Horny Goat Weed extract is 500–1,000 mg per day.

Ginseng (*Panax ginseng*)

Panax Ginseng, also known as **Korean Ginseng**, is one of the most widely studied herbs for sexual health. It has been shown to improve libido, increase energy levels, and support overall sexual performance. Ginseng works as an adaptogen, helping the body adapt to stress and reducing fatigue, both of which can negatively impact sexual health. Additionally, it increases **nitric oxide** production, promoting improved blood flow to the genital area and enhancing sexual function. Ginseng is particularly beneficial for individuals experiencing low libido due to stress, exhaustion, or hormonal imbalances.

- **How to Use:** Ginseng is typically available in capsule, tablet, powder, or liquid extract form.
- **Dosage:** The typical recommended dose for Panax Ginseng is 200–400 mg of standardized extract per day.

Ashwagandha (*Withania somnifera*)

Ashwagandha is an adaptogenic herb that helps reduce stress, balance hormones, and improve energy, all of which play an essential role in maintaining a healthy libido. Chronic stress and imbalances in **cortisol** levels are often linked to a reduced sex drive, and Ashwagandha helps to regulate stress hormones while enhancing overall vitality. This herb has been shown to improve sexual function, increase fertility in both men and women, and enhance sexual desire by balancing the body's hormonal system.

- **How to Use:** Ashwagandha is available in capsules, powders, or tinctures. It can also be added to teas and smoothies.
- **Dosage:** The typical dose of Ashwagandha extract is 300–600 mg per day, often divided into two doses.

Damiana (*Turnera diffusa*)

Damiana is a traditional herb known for its aphrodisiac properties. Native to Central and South America, Damiana has been used for centuries to improve sexual desire and performance. It works by increasing blood flow to the sexual organs, stimulating the nervous system, and balancing hormones. Damiana is especially beneficial for individuals suffering from low libido, stress-related sexual dysfunction, or menopausal changes. It also helps to enhance overall mood and energy, which can improve sexual vitality.

- **How to Use:** Damiana is available in capsules, teas, or tinctures.
- **Dosage:** A typical dose is 400–800 mg of Damiana extract per day, or 1–2 cups of Damiana tea.

Shatavari (*Asparagus racemosus*)

Shatavari is an important herb in Ayurvedic medicine, particularly for women's reproductive health. It is known to support hormonal balance, improve fertility, and increase libido. Shatavari works by nourishing the **female reproductive system**, promoting healthy ovulation, and supporting the body's ability to cope with stress. It is also used to increase sexual desire, alleviate symptoms of PMS and menopause, and enhance overall vitality. While primarily used by women, Shatavari can also support male sexual health by balancing overall energy and vitality.

- **How to Use**: Shatavari is typically consumed in powder or capsule form. It can also be made into a tea.
- **Dosage**: A typical dose of Shatavari powder is 1–2 teaspoons per day, or 500–1,000 mg of Shatavari extract.

Saffron (*Crocus sativus*)

Saffron, the spice derived from the flower of **Crocus sativus**, is not only a prized culinary ingredient but also a potent herb for enhancing libido and sexual function. Research has shown that Saffron can increase sexual desire, improve erectile function, and boost overall sexual satisfaction. Saffron's ability to balance **serotonin** and **dopamine** levels helps to reduce stress and anxiety, both of which are often significant contributors to low libido. Additionally, Saffron has antioxidant properties that support overall reproductive health.

- **How to Use**: Saffron is available in powdered form or as a supplement.
- **Dosage**: A typical dose of Saffron extract is 30 mg per day, or a pinch (around 0.5–1 gram) of saffron powder in food or tea.

Yohimbe (*Pausinystalia johimbe*)

Yohimbe is an herb derived from the bark of the **Yohimbe tree**, native to Central Africa. It has long been used to treat erectile dysfunction and enhance libido. Yohimbe works by increasing blood flow to the genitals, improving circulation, and stimulating the release of **nitric oxide**, which is essential for achieving and maintaining erections. It also helps to stimulate nerve function and reduce the symptoms of sexual dysfunction caused by stress or anxiety.

- **How to Use**: Yohimbe is available in capsules, tablets, and tinctures.
- **Dosage**: The typical recommended dose is 5–10 mg of Yohimbe extract per day. However, Yohimbe should be used with caution, as it can cause side effects in some individuals (such as anxiety, high blood pressure, and heart palpitations). It's important to consult a healthcare provider before use.

Eye Health Herbs

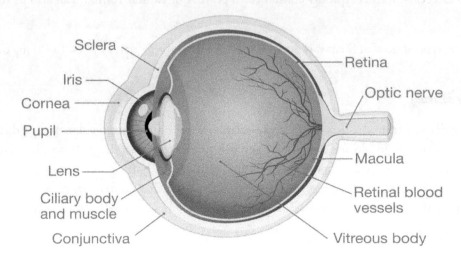

Our eyes are essential to how we interact with the world, yet they are often overlooked when it comes to overall health and wellness. Factors such as aging, environmental stress, digital screen exposure, poor nutrition, and even genetics can affect the health of our eyes and lead to various vision problems. Fortunately, nature offers a wide range of herbs that can support eye health, improve vision, and protect the eyes from damage caused by oxidative stress, inflammation, and other harmful factors.

Herbs for eye health work in various ways—some are rich in antioxidants that protect the eyes from oxidative damage, while others enhance blood circulation to the eyes or support healthy vision by providing essential nutrients. Many of these herbs have been used for centuries in traditional medicine systems to maintain optimal eye health, alleviate discomfort, and improve visual function.

Bilberry (*Vaccinium myrtillus*)

Bilberry is one of the most well-known herbs for eye health. It is rich in **anthocyanins**, a powerful group of antioxidants that help improve blood circulation to the eyes, strengthen blood vessels, and protect the retina from oxidative stress. Bilberry is particularly beneficial for individuals experiencing **night blindness**, **macular degeneration**, and **eye strain**. Studies have shown that Bilberry can enhance vision, reduce eye fatigue, and support long-term eye health by protecting against UV damage.

- **How to Use:** Bilberry is commonly consumed as a supplement (capsules or tablets) or in the form of dried fruit. It can also be brewed into tea.

- **Dosage:** A typical dose of Bilberry extract is 80–160 mg per day, often standardized to 25% anthocyanins.

Eyebright (*Euphrasia officinalis*)

Eyebright has been traditionally used for centuries to treat a variety of eye conditions, including conjunctivitis, eye irritation, and eye fatigue. This herb is known for its **anti-inflammatory** and **antiseptic** properties, making it particularly effective for soothing eye discomfort, reducing redness, and relieving dryness. Eyebright is also believed to support overall eye health by improving circulation to the eyes and reducing swelling. It is commonly used to address issues like **sinus-related eye problems** and **allergic reactions**.

- **How to Use**: Eyebright is available as a tincture, capsule, or as an herbal tea. It can also be used topically in the form of a compress for sore or inflamed eyes.
- **Dosage**: For internal use, 1–2 teaspoons of Eyebright tincture or tea can be taken up to three times per day. For external use, Eyebright can be soaked in water and used as an eye wash or compress.

Lutein and Zeaxanthin (from Marigold and Spinach)

Lutein and Zeaxanthin are carotenoids that play a crucial role in protecting the eyes from harmful **blue light** and oxidative stress. These antioxidants are naturally found in high concentrations in the **macula** of the eye, where they help filter out blue light and prevent damage to the retina. They also protect against age-related macular degeneration (AMD), cataracts, and other degenerative eye diseases. While Lutein and Zeaxanthin are found in foods like **spinach, kale,** and **egg yolks, marigold flowers** are an excellent source of these important carotenoids.

- **How to Use**: Lutein and Zeaxanthin are commonly available as standalone supplements or in combination with other eye health nutrients (like Vitamin C and Zinc). You can also consume them naturally by adding spinach, kale, and marigold flower extract to your diet.
- **Dosage**: A typical dosage for Lutein is 10–20 mg per day, and for Zeaxanthin, 2–4 mg per day, often as part of a comprehensive eye health formula.

Ginkgo Biloba (*Ginkgo biloba*)

Ginkgo Biloba is widely known for its ability to improve blood circulation and enhance cognitive function, but it also offers significant benefits for eye health. By improving circulation to the eyes, Ginkgo Biloba helps to nourish the delicate blood vessels in the retina, reduce eye fatigue, and support healthy vision. Ginkgo is also a powerful antioxidant that helps to protect the eyes from oxidative damage caused by free radicals, thus promoting long-term eye health and reducing the risk of cataracts and age-related macular degeneration.

- **How to Use**: Ginkgo Biloba is available in capsules, tablets, or as a liquid extract.
- **Dosage**: The recommended dosage of Ginkgo Biloba extract is 120–240 mg per day, often divided into two doses.

Turmeric (*Curcuma longa*)

Turmeric, with its active compound **curcumin**, is a potent anti-inflammatory and antioxidant herb that supports eye health. Curcumin helps reduce inflammation in the eyes, which can be beneficial for conditions such as **uveitis** (inflammation of the eye) and **dry eye syndrome**. Additionally, curcumin has been shown to protect against retinal damage and oxidative stress, reducing the risk of cataracts and macular degeneration.

Its ability to support the body's natural detoxification processes also plays a role in maintaining overall eye health.

- **How to Use:** Turmeric can be consumed as a supplement, in cooking, or brewed into a tea. For enhanced absorption, it is often combined with black pepper or healthy fats.

- **Dosage:** The typical dosage of curcumin extract is 500–1,000 mg per day.

Black Currant (*Ribes nigrum*)

Black Currant is a rich source of **anthocyanins**, similar to Bilberry, and has powerful antioxidant and anti-inflammatory properties that support eye health. Studies have shown that Black Currant extract can improve **night vision**, reduce eye strain, and protect the eyes from the damaging effects of oxidative stress. It also has potential benefits for individuals with **glaucoma** or **diabetic retinopathy**, as it helps to improve circulation and reduce intraocular pressure (IOP).

- **How to Use:** Black Currant is available in capsules, as an extract, or in the form of juice.

- **Dosage:** The typical dose of Black Currant extract is 200–500 mg per day.

Carrot (*Daucus carota*)

Carrots are one of the most well-known foods for eye health due to their high content of **beta-carotene**, a precursor to **Vitamin A**, which is essential for maintaining good vision. Vitamin A supports the **retina**, helping to convert light into nerve signals that the brain interprets as images. A deficiency in Vitamin A can lead to night blindness and other vision issues. Consuming carrots regularly supports healthy vision, particularly in low-light conditions, and helps to maintain the overall health of the eye structures.

- **How to Use:** Carrots can be eaten raw, juiced, or added to meals. Carrot juice or puree is an excellent source of beta-carotene.

- **Dosage:** Consuming 1–2 medium-sized carrots daily provides a good dose of beta-carotene.

Saffron (*Crocus sativus*)

Saffron, the prized spice derived from the **Crocus sativus** flower, has been found to support eye health by improving vision and protecting against conditions like macular degeneration. The active compounds in saffron, particularly **crocin** and **safranal**, have been shown to enhance retinal health, reduce oxidative damage, and improve blood circulation to the eyes. Research indicates that saffron can help improve visual acuity, especially in older adults, and protect the eyes from damage caused by aging and UV exposure.

- **How to Use:** Saffron can be consumed as a supplement or added to food and beverages, such as teas, soups, or rice dishes.

- **Dosage:** A typical dose of saffron extract is 20–30 mg per day.

Rosehip (*Rosa canina*)

Rosehip is a rich source of **Vitamin C**, a powerful antioxidant that helps protect the eyes from oxidative damage and supports overall eye health. Vitamin C plays a key role in the health of the **cornea** and **retina**, as well as in the prevention of cataracts. The high antioxidant content in Rosehip also helps to reduce inflammation in the eyes and improve blood circulation, which can alleviate symptoms of eye strain and fatigue.

- **How to Use:** Rosehip is available as a supplement, tea, or in the form of oil for topical use.
- **Dosage:** A typical dose of Rosehip extract is 500–1,000 mg per day.

Antiseptic & Healing Herbs

In our daily lives, cuts, scrapes, bruises, and infections are common occurrences. While modern medicine has provided effective treatments for these issues, nature also offers a wealth of powerful herbs that have antiseptic and healing properties. These herbs can be used to treat minor wounds, prevent infection, and promote faster recovery, all while being gentle on the skin.

Antiseptic and healing herbs are known for their ability to cleanse wounds, kill harmful pathogens, reduce inflammation, and encourage tissue regeneration. Many of these herbs have been used for centuries in traditional medicine for their ability to support the body's natural healing processes. By integrating these herbs into your first aid routine or daily skincare regimen, you can enhance your body's natural ability to heal while preventing infections and promoting skin health.

Aloe Vera (*Aloe barbadensis miller*)

Aloe Vera is perhaps the most well-known herb for skin healing and wound care. Its gel, extracted from the thick leaves of the plant, is packed with **antibacterial**, **anti-inflammatory**, and **moisturizing** compounds. Aloe Vera promotes healing by reducing pain, inflammation, and redness while keeping the skin hydrated. It also contains **polysaccharides** that support tissue regeneration and **glycoproteins** that help to soothe irritated skin. Aloe Vera is particularly beneficial for burns, cuts, abrasions, and insect bites.

- **How to Use:** Aloe Vera gel can be applied directly to the affected area or used in creams and lotions. Fresh gel can be extracted from the plant's leaves for immediate use.
- **Dosage:** Apply Aloe Vera gel 2–3 times per day until the wound or irritation heals.

Calendula (*Calendula officinalis*)

Calendula, also known as **marigold**, is renowned for its healing and soothing properties. This vibrant yellow-orange flower has natural **antiseptic**, **anti-inflammatory**, and **antifungal** effects, making it a great remedy for skin infections, minor cuts, and scrapes. Calendula enhances wound healing by promoting tissue regeneration, reducing swelling, and preventing infection. It also helps to ease irritation and redness in conditions like eczema and dermatitis.

- **How to Use:** Calendula is commonly found in creams, ointments, and oils, but can also be used in a tea for external applications. A diluted calendula tincture can also be applied to the skin.
- **Dosage:** For topical use, apply Calendula cream or ointment to the affected area 2–3 times a day.

Lavender (*Lavandula angustifolia*)

Lavender is not only cherished for its calming fragrance but also for its antiseptic and healing properties. **Lavender essential oil** is particularly effective in treating small cuts, burns, insect bites, and skin irritations due to its **antibacterial, antiviral**, and **anti-inflammatory** effects. Lavender also promotes skin regeneration and helps to reduce scarring. It can be used to disinfect minor wounds and speed up the healing process.

- **How to Use**: Lavender oil should be diluted in a carrier oil (such as coconut oil or olive oil) before applying to the skin. A few drops can also be added to creams or ointments.
- **Dosage**: For topical use, apply diluted lavender oil to the affected area up to 2–3 times a day.

Tea Tree Oil (*Melaleuca alternifolia*)

Tea Tree Oil is a powerhouse herb known for its **antiseptic, antifungal**, and **antiviral** properties. It is particularly useful in treating skin conditions like acne, athlete's foot, fungal infections, and minor cuts. Tea Tree Oil works by killing harmful microorganisms, reducing inflammation, and promoting faster wound healing. It's also commonly used in natural remedies for **ingrown hairs, shingles**, and **cold sores**.

- **How to Use**: Tea Tree Oil must always be diluted with a carrier oil (such as jojoba or olive oil) before being applied directly to the skin. It can also be added to ointments and creams for localized use.
- **Dosage**: Use a few drops of diluted Tea Tree Oil on the affected area 2–3 times per day, depending on the severity of the condition.

Comfrey (*Symphytum officinale*)

Comfrey is a highly effective herb for promoting healing and reducing pain in damaged tissues. Its **allantoin** content encourages the growth of new skin cells and tissue regeneration, making it ideal for healing cuts, bruises, sprains, and fractures. Comfrey has been traditionally used to treat burns, wounds, and **muscle injuries** due to its ability to reduce inflammation and stimulate the healing process. However, it should be used with caution on broken skin, as it can potentially cause skin irritation if used improperly.

- **How to Use**: Comfrey can be applied topically as a cream, ointment, or poultice. The dried root or leaves can also be infused into oil for topical use.
- **Dosage**: Apply a thin layer of Comfrey cream or ointment to the affected area 1–2 times a day.

Echinacea (*Echinacea purpurea*)

Echinacea is widely recognized for its immune-boosting properties, but it also has notable antiseptic and healing effects when applied topically. Echinacea can be used to treat minor wounds, skin infections, and **inflammatory conditions** like eczema and acne. Its **anti-inflammatory** and **antibacterial** properties help reduce redness, swelling, and pain, while stimulating the skin's natural healing process. Echinacea also supports the body's immune response, helping to fight off infection at the wound site.

- **How to Use**: Echinacea is typically used as a tincture, cream, or oil. It can also be brewed into a tea for internal use to support immune function.

- **Dosage:** For topical use, apply Echinacea cream or ointment to the affected area 2–3 times daily.

Plantain (*Plantago major*)

Plantain is a common herb with impressive healing abilities, particularly for skin wounds and inflammation. Known for its **antiseptic, anti-inflammatory**, and **analgesic** properties, Plantain helps to clean wounds, reduce swelling, and alleviate pain. It is particularly effective for **insect bites**, **stings**, **scrapes**, and **cuts**. Plantain has also been used traditionally to treat **skin rashes**, **blisters**, and even **poison ivy**.

- **How to Use:** Fresh Plantain leaves can be crushed and applied directly to the skin to treat wounds. Plantain is also available in ointments, tinctures, and creams.
- **Dosage:** Apply fresh Plantain poultices to the wound, or use Plantain-based creams 2–3 times a day.

St. John's Wort (*Hypericum perforatum*)

St. John's Wort is a well-known herb for mood and nerve support, but it is also incredibly effective in healing wounds and burns. It contains **hypericin**, a compound that possesses **antiseptic** and **anti-inflammatory** properties. St. John's Wort is especially useful for **nerve pain** and injuries, such as **burns**, **cuts**, and **bruises**. It is often used in treating **nerve-related pain** (such as from shingles) and to reduce scar tissue after healing.

- **How to Use:** St. John's Wort is often used in oil form, where the flowers are infused in a carrier oil like olive oil. It can be applied topically as a salve or ointment.
- **Dosage:** Apply St. John's Wort oil or salve to affected areas 2–3 times a day.

Myrrh (*Commiphora wightii*)

Myrrh is an ancient resin known for its potent **antiseptic** and **anti-inflammatory** properties. It is particularly effective for healing **gums**, **mouth ulcers**, **wounds**, and **skin infections**. Myrrh helps to disinfect and promote healing in damaged tissues while reducing swelling and pain. It also has **antifungal** and **antiviral** properties, making it useful for treating infections such as athlete's foot and ringworm.

- **How to Use:** Myrrh is most commonly used as an essential oil, diluted in a carrier oil for topical application, or as a tincture.
- **Dosage:** Use diluted Myrrh oil on wounds and infections 2–3 times per day.

Antidepressant & Mood-Boosting Herbs

In today's fast-paced world, it's common for many people to experience periods of stress, anxiety, and even feelings of sadness or low energy. While traditional medicine provides solutions for these issues, many are turning to nature for holistic support. Herbs that act as natural antidepressants and mood boosters have been used for centuries across cultures to improve mental well-being, enhance emotional balance, and promote relaxation.

These herbs work by supporting the nervous system, regulating key hormones like serotonin and dopamine, and reducing stress or inflammation, all of which contribute to better mood and emotional stability. Whether you're dealing with mild mood swings or looking for natural ways to support your mental health, these herbs offer powerful, plant-based alternatives to pharmaceutical treatments.

St. John's Wort (*Hypericum perforatum*)

St. John's Wort is perhaps the most widely recognized herb for enhancing mood and alleviating symptoms of **depression** and **anxiety**. It has been extensively studied and shown to work similarly to conventional antidepressants by influencing the levels of **serotonin, dopamine**, and **norepinephrine** in the brain. This herb is particularly effective for mild to moderate depression and is commonly used to improve mood, reduce feelings of sadness, and promote mental clarity.

- **How it works**: St. John's Wort contains active compounds like **hypericin** and **hyperforin**, which help balance neurotransmitters, thus boosting mood and relieving symptoms of depression. It also has mild **anti-inflammatory** effects, which may help calm the nervous system.
- **How to use**: St. John's Wort can be taken as a tea, tincture, or in capsule form. The oil extract is also used in topical applications for its calming effects on the skin.
- **Dosage**: Standardized extracts (containing 0.3% hypericin) are usually taken in doses of 300–900 mg per day, divided into 1–3 doses.

Rhodiola (*Rhodiola rosea*)

Rhodiola, also known as **golden root**, is an adaptogenic herb that helps the body adapt to stress while promoting a balanced mood. Rhodiola works by balancing the levels of key neurotransmitters such as **serotonin, dopamine**, and **norepinephrine**, while also helping to **reduce cortisol**—the stress hormone. This herb is especially beneficial for those suffering from **stress-induced fatigue**, burnout, and anxiety. It enhances both physical and mental endurance, which can be crucial when dealing with emotional or psychological strain.

- **How it works**: Rhodiola boosts energy, reduces stress, and improves cognitive function. It can improve mood by promoting a better stress response, and it has mild **antidepressant** and **anxiolytic** effects.
- **How to use**: Rhodiola is most commonly consumed in capsule or tincture form, and it can also be found in some energy drinks and supplements.
- **Dosage**: The typical dosage is between 200–400 mg per day, depending on the concentration of the extract.

Ashwagandha (*Withania somnifera*)

Ashwagandha, a revered herb in Ayurvedic medicine, is known for its powerful **adaptogenic** properties. It helps the body manage stress and anxiety by regulating the **HPA axis** (hypothalamic-pituitary-adrenal axis) and lowering **cortisol** levels. This herb has a calming effect on the nervous system, which helps relieve feelings of tension, irritability, and anxiety. Ashwagandha also boosts energy and stamina, making it ideal for combating both physical and mental fatigue associated with depression.

- **How it works**: By regulating cortisol and supporting the adrenal glands, Ashwagandha helps the body adapt to stress. It also enhances the function of the **serotonergic** system, which plays a key role in regulating mood.
- **How to use**: Ashwagandha is typically taken in powder, capsule, or tincture form.
- **Dosage**: Standardized extracts (containing 5% withanolides) are typically taken in doses of 300–600 mg per day.

Lavender (*Lavandula angustifolia*)

Lavender is widely known for its calming and relaxing properties, and it has also been shown to improve mood and reduce symptoms of anxiety and depression. The active compounds in lavender, particularly **linalool**, interact with the **GABA receptors** in the brain, helping to induce relaxation and reduce nervous tension. Lavender is especially helpful for those dealing with **insomnia**, **restlessness**, or stress-induced emotional imbalances.

- **How it works**: Lavender works by modulating the nervous system and reducing the symptoms of stress, anxiety, and mild depression. It is often used in aromatherapy to promote relaxation and emotional well-being.
- **How to use**: Lavender can be used as an essential oil (in aromatherapy), in teas, or in capsule form. Lavender oil can also be applied topically, diluted in a carrier oil, to relieve anxiety or stress.
- **Dosage**: When using lavender essential oil, diffuse it for 20–30 minutes daily or use 2–3 drops diluted in a carrier oil for topical use.

Lemon Balm (*Melissa officinalis*)

Lemon Balm, a member of the mint family, is known for its mild sedative and mood-boosting effects. It helps reduce anxiety, promote relaxation, and support emotional well-being. Lemon Balm works by enhancing the effects of **GABA** (gamma-aminobutyric acid), a neurotransmitter that inhibits nerve activity, helping to calm the mind and body. It is often used to improve mood, reduce anxiety, and relieve symptoms of **nervous tension**.

- **How it works**: Lemon Balm improves mood by calming the nervous system, and it also has mild **antidepressant** and **anxiolytic** effects. It can be particularly useful for people with **insomnia** or **mild anxiety**.
- **How to use**: Lemon Balm can be consumed as a tea, tincture, or in capsule form.
- **Dosage**: For the best results, take 300–500 mg of standardized Lemon Balm extract, or drink 1–2 cups of Lemon Balm tea daily.

Holy Basil (Tulsi) (*Ocimum sanctum*)

Holy Basil, also known as **Tulsi**, is a revered herb in Ayurvedic medicine and a powerful adaptogen. It helps reduce the physical and mental impact of stress, anxiety, and depression. Holy Basil works by balancing **cortisol** levels and supporting the body's natural response to emotional and physical strain. It also has antioxidant and anti-inflammatory properties that help restore balance to the nervous system, boosting overall mental clarity and emotional resilience.

- **How it works:** Holy Basil supports the adrenal glands, promotes mental clarity, and reduces the effects of stress. Its **adaptogenic** properties help stabilize mood and improve emotional resilience.
- **How to use:** Holy Basil can be taken as a tea, in capsule form, or as a tincture.
- **Dosage:** A typical dosage of Holy Basil extract is 300–500 mg per day, or 1–2 cups of Tulsi tea.

Passionflower (*Passiflora incarnata*)

Passionflower is another excellent herb for promoting relaxation and reducing anxiety. It has a **calming effect** on the nervous system and has been used to treat insomnia, **nervous tension**, and **stress-related anxiety**. Passionflower works by increasing the levels of **GABA** in the brain, which helps to calm overactive neurons and reduce feelings of restlessness. It is especially helpful for people who suffer from anxiety-related insomnia.

- **How it works:** Passionflower helps to reduce symptoms of anxiety and depression by promoting relaxation, improving sleep, and balancing neurotransmitters in the brain.
- **How to use:** Passionflower can be consumed as a tea, tincture, or in capsule form.
- **Dosage:** For best results, take 250–500 mg of Passionflower extract or drink 1–2 cups of Passionflower tea daily.

Ginseng (*Panax ginseng*)

Ginseng, a well-known **adaptogen**, helps to enhance physical and mental energy while reducing symptoms of fatigue and depression. It supports the adrenal glands and helps the body adapt to stress, thereby improving mood and emotional stability. Ginseng also has mild **antidepressant** properties and can increase mental clarity, focus, and overall well-being.

- **How it works:** Ginseng balances energy levels, reduces fatigue, and enhances mood by improving blood circulation to the brain and increasing levels of neurotransmitters like **serotonin** and **dopamine**.
- **How to use:** Ginseng is available in capsule, extract, or tea form.
- **Dosage:** Standardized extracts of Ginseng are typically taken in doses of 100–400 mg per day.

Menstrual Health & Women's Reproductive Health Herbs

Women's reproductive health is a vital and often complex aspect of overall well-being, encompassing a range of functions from the menstrual cycle to fertility, and from hormonal balance to menopause. Traditional herbal remedies have long been used to support these functions, helping women navigate the various stages of life with comfort and ease. Whether managing painful menstruation, irregular cycles, or seeking support for fertility, herbs can offer effective, natural solutions that complement conventional care.

Herbal remedies for menstrual health and women's reproductive health work by balancing hormones, alleviating discomfort, and supporting the body's natural processes. Many of these herbs have adaptogenic, anti-inflammatory, and antispasmodic properties, making them highly effective for addressing common menstrual issues, including **cramps**, **PMS**, and **heavy periods**. Additionally, they play a key role in enhancing fertility, regulating cycles, and easing the transition into menopause.

Red Clover (*Trifolium pratense*)

Red Clover is a herb well-known for its ability to support women's reproductive health, particularly in regulating the menstrual cycle and supporting hormonal balance. Rich in **phytoestrogens**, compounds that mimic the action of estrogen in the body, Red Clover can help alleviate symptoms associated with hormonal fluctuations, including **PMS** and **menopausal symptoms**. It also has **anti-inflammatory** and **detoxifying** properties, promoting overall reproductive wellness.

- **How it works**: Red Clover helps to regulate estrogen levels and support the endocrine system, making it particularly beneficial for women experiencing hormonal imbalances. It is also commonly used to ease menstrual cramps and reduce hot flashes during menopause.
- **How to use**: Red Clover is typically consumed as a tea, tincture, or in capsule form.
- **Dosage**: For tea, drink 1–2 cups daily; for capsules or tinctures, follow the recommended dosage on the product label, generally 300–500 mg per day.

Dong Quai (*Angelica sinensis*)

Known as the "female ginseng," **Dong Quai** has been used in traditional Chinese medicine for centuries to support menstrual health and women's reproductive function. This herb is prized for its ability to **regulate menstrual cycles**, relieve **menstrual cramps**, and support overall uterine health. It contains compounds that help balance estrogen levels, reduce inflammation, and improve circulation, making it particularly useful for women suffering from **irregular periods** or **painful menstruation**.

- **How it works**: Dong Quai works by toning the uterus, improving blood circulation, and balancing hormones. It can also help ease the discomfort associated with PMS and promote a more regular cycle.
- **How to use**: Dong Quai is typically taken as a tincture, capsule, or in tea form.
- **Dosage**: Standard doses range from 500–1000 mg per day in capsule form or 1–2 teaspoons of tincture per day. For tea, drink 1–2 cups daily.

Chaste Tree Berry (Vitex) (*Vitex agnus-castus*)

Vitex, commonly known as **Chaste Tree Berry**, is one of the most well-known herbs for supporting menstrual health and balancing female hormones. It works primarily by stimulating the pituitary gland to regulate the production of **luteinizing hormone (LH)**, which in turn helps balance the ratio of estrogen to progesterone in the body. This action is particularly helpful for women experiencing **irregular cycles**, **PMS**, **mood swings**, and **breast tenderness**.

- **How it works**: Vitex is an excellent herb for restoring hormonal balance and supporting the **luteal phase** of the menstrual cycle. It is often used to treat symptoms of **PMS** and to support fertility.
- **How to use**: Chaste Tree Berry can be taken as a capsule, tincture, or in tea form.
- **Dosage**: Typically, 400–500 mg of Chaste Tree Berry extract per day, or 1–2 teaspoons of tincture daily.

Cramp Bark (*Viburnum opulus*)

As the name suggests, **Cramp Bark** is especially effective for alleviating **menstrual cramps** and **abdominal discomfort** associated with menstruation. It has **antispasmodic** and **anti-inflammatory** properties that help relax the muscles of the uterus and reduce cramping. Cramp Bark is also beneficial for **pelvic pain, lower back pain**, and **muscle tension**, providing natural relief during menstruation.

- **How it works**: Cramp Bark works by relaxing smooth muscle tissues in the uterus, thereby reducing spasms and easing discomfort associated with menstrual cramps.
- **How to use**: Cramp Bark is often taken as a tincture, tea, or in capsule form.
- **Dosage**: The typical dosage is 1–2 teaspoons of Cramp Bark tincture, or 400–500 mg of the extract, taken 2–3 times daily during the menstrual cycle.

Black Cohosh (*Actaea racemosa*)

Black Cohosh is a powerful herb that has been traditionally used to ease **menopausal symptoms** such as hot flashes, night sweats, and mood swings. It can also be used to manage **PMS** and **menstrual cramps**. Black Cohosh works by interacting with the **estrogen receptors** in the body, providing a mild estrogenic effect, which helps balance hormonal fluctuations during menstruation and menopause.

- **How it works**: Black Cohosh helps modulate estrogen activity, thereby easing symptoms of hormone imbalance. It is particularly useful for managing symptoms of **perimenopause** and **menopause**, as well as for reducing cramps and menstrual discomfort.
- **How to use**: Black Cohosh is available in tincture, capsule, and tablet forms.
- **Dosage**: The typical dosage is 40–80 mg per day of standardized Black Cohosh extract, or 1–2 teaspoons of tincture daily.

Raspberry Leaf (*Rubus idaeus*)

Raspberry Leaf is a well-known herb that has long been used to support **uterine health**, regulate **menstrual cycles**, and ease **labor pains**. Rich in **vitamins** and **minerals**, especially **iron** and **calcium**, Raspberry Leaf helps tone the uterus and supports the menstrual flow. It is also valuable for relieving symptoms of **PMS**, such as bloating and irritability.

- **How it works**: Raspberry Leaf helps to tone and strengthen the uterus, making it particularly beneficial for women experiencing **heavy periods** or **cramps**. It also promotes overall **reproductive health** by improving circulation and providing essential nutrients.

- **How to use**: Raspberry Leaf is most commonly consumed as a tea but is also available in capsules or tincture form.
- **Dosage**: For tea, drink 1–3 cups daily, or follow the recommended dosage on capsule products, typically 500–1000 mg per day.

Evening Primrose Oil (*Oenothera biennis*)

Evening Primrose Oil is a well-known supplement used to alleviate **PMS** and balance hormones. The oil is rich in **gamma-linolenic acid (GLA)**, an essential fatty acid that helps reduce **inflammation**, support hormonal balance, and promote overall reproductive health. Evening Primrose Oil is often used to treat **breast tenderness**, **mood swings**, and **irritability** associated with PMS.

- **How it works**: Evening Primrose Oil helps to regulate **prostaglandin** production, which can reduce inflammation and muscle cramping during menstruation. It also helps to balance estrogen and progesterone levels, providing relief from hormonal fluctuations.
- **How to use**: Evening Primrose Oil is typically taken in capsule form.
- **Dosage**: A common dose is 500–1000 mg per day of Evening Primrose Oil.

Aloe Vera (*Aloe barbadensis miller*)

Aloe Vera is often associated with skin care, but it also offers significant benefits for **reproductive health**. Aloe Vera has **anti-inflammatory**, **detoxifying**, and **soothing** properties, making it beneficial for women experiencing **heavy menstrual bleeding** or **irregular cycles**. It also supports the digestive system and enhances the body's ability to eliminate toxins, which can improve overall hormone regulation.

- **How it works**: Aloe Vera promotes detoxification and helps reduce inflammation in the body, supporting overall menstrual health. It also contains **gibberellins**, which can help regulate hormone levels and encourage healthy uterine function.
- **How to use**: Aloe Vera juice or gel can be consumed internally or applied topically to soothe skin irritations associated with menstruation.
- **Dosage**: Drink 1–2 tablespoons of Aloe Vera juice daily, or apply Aloe Vera gel as needed for skin relief.

Anti-Cancer & Tumor-Fighting Herbs

Cancer, a complex and often devastating disease, has long been a challenge in both conventional and complementary medicine. While traditional treatments such as chemotherapy, radiation, and surgery are standard methods for combating cancer, many individuals seek additional support from nature's pharmacy to boost their immune system, reduce inflammation, and inhibit tumor growth. Herbal remedies, with their bioactive compounds, have gained significant attention for their potential to fight cancer, prevent metastasis, and improve quality of life during cancer treatment.

Numerous herbs contain potent **antioxidants**, **anti-inflammatory**, and **anticarcinogenic** properties, which can help support the body's natural defense mechanisms. These herbs work in a variety of ways, from boosting the immune system to interfering with cancer cell growth and inhibiting tumor formation. While they are not intended to replace medical treatments, they can be used as complementary therapies to support overall health, strengthen the body's resistance, and enhance the efficacy of conventional cancer treatments.

Turmeric (*Curcuma longa*)

Turmeric, the golden-yellow spice that's a staple in many cuisines, has long been known for its powerful **anti-inflammatory**, **antioxidant**, and **anticancer** properties. The active compound in turmeric, **curcumin**, has been extensively studied for its ability to inhibit the growth of cancer cells, prevent metastasis, and reduce the side effects of cancer treatments like chemotherapy.

- **How it works**: Curcumin works by targeting several biological pathways involved in cancer development, including inflammation, oxidative stress, and apoptosis (programmed cell death). It has been shown to block the activation of key molecules that promote tumor growth and spread, and it may help prevent the transformation of healthy cells into cancerous ones.

- **How to use**: Turmeric can be consumed as a spice in food, in capsule form, or as a tincture. For enhanced absorption, it is often paired with **black pepper**, which contains **piperine**, a compound that improves curcumin's bioavailability.

- **Dosage**: Standardized turmeric extracts with 95% curcumin can be taken in doses of 500–2000 mg per day, often divided into 1–3 doses.

Green Tea (*Camellia sinensis*)

Green Tea is celebrated for its numerous health benefits, particularly its **antioxidant** properties, which come from high concentrations of **catechins**. One of the most powerful catechins, **epigallocatechin gallate (EGCG)**, has been shown to have potent **anticancer** effects by preventing cancer cell proliferation, inducing apoptosis, and inhibiting the formation of new blood vessels that tumors need to grow.

- **How it works**: EGCG in green tea blocks specific enzymes that promote cancer cell division and metastasis. It has also been shown to enhance the effects of chemotherapy and radiation, making it a valuable ally in cancer treatment. Additionally, it can reduce inflammation and oxidative damage, which are linked to cancer development.

- **How to use**: Green tea can be consumed as a hot or iced beverage, or in capsule or extract form.

- **Dosage**: To benefit from the cancer-fighting effects, aim for 3–5 cups of green tea per day or 300–500 mg of green tea extract (EGCG) daily.

Milk Thistle (*Silybum marianum*)

Milk Thistle, known for its liver-protective properties, has shown promise as an anti-cancer herb due to its active compound **silymarin**. Silymarin is a potent **antioxidant** and **anti-inflammatory** agent that has been studied for its ability to protect healthy cells from damage while inhibiting the growth of cancer cells, particularly in the liver, breast, and prostate.

- **How it works**: Silymarin works by blocking the formation of free radicals, which contribute to cancer development. It also enhances liver function, helping the body detoxify and eliminate harmful substances that could promote cancer. In addition, silymarin may help prevent tumor growth and reduce the toxicity of chemotherapy.
- **How to use**: Milk Thistle is commonly consumed in capsule, tablet, or tincture form.
- **Dosage**: Standardized Milk Thistle extract (containing 70–80% silymarin) is typically taken in doses of 140–400 mg per day.

Ginger (*Zingiber officinale*)

Ginger, a widely used spice with **anti-inflammatory** and **antioxidant** properties, has demonstrated significant potential in the fight against cancer. It has been shown to reduce inflammation, inhibit cancer cell proliferation, and even induce apoptosis in cancer cells. Ginger is particularly beneficial for those undergoing cancer treatment, as it can help reduce nausea, a common side effect of chemotherapy.

- **How it works**: The active compounds in ginger, such as **gingerol, shogaol**, and **paradols**, have been found to suppress tumor growth by modulating several signaling pathways involved in cancer progression. Ginger can also help reduce the **inflammatory cytokines** that contribute to cancer development.
- **How to use**: Ginger can be consumed fresh, in teas, as a supplement, or as a powdered spice.
- **Dosage**: Typical dosages range from 500–1000 mg of ginger extract per day or 1–2 grams of fresh ginger root, taken in divided doses.

Astragalus (*Astragalus membranaceus*)

Astragalus, an adaptogenic herb used in traditional Chinese medicine, is well-known for its immune-boosting properties. It helps enhance the body's natural defense system, which is critical for fighting cancer. Astragalus contains **polysaccharides** that stimulate the production of **T-cells** and **macrophages**, vital components of the immune system.

- **How it works**: By boosting the immune system and promoting healthy cell function, Astragalus has shown potential in slowing the progression of cancer, preventing recurrence, and improving overall vitality during cancer treatment. It is also thought to reduce the side effects of chemotherapy and radiation.
- **How to use**: Astragalus is available as a capsule, powder, or tincture. It can also be brewed as a tea.
- **Dosage**: The typical dose is 500–1500 mg per day of Astragalus extract or 1–2 teaspoons of the dried root, taken 2–3 times daily.

Graviola (Soursop) (*Annona muricata*)

Graviola, also known as **Soursop**, is a tropical fruit that has gained popularity for its potential **anticancer** properties. It contains compounds known as **acetogenins**, which have been shown to inhibit the growth of cancer cells by selectively targeting and destroying malignant cells while leaving healthy cells unharmed. Early research suggests Graviola may be effective against several types of cancer, including **breast**, **prostate**, **liver**, and **pancreatic** cancers.

- **How it works**: Graviola's acetogenins disrupt the mitochondrial function in cancer cells, leading to cell death. The compounds also have **antioxidant** and **anti-inflammatory** effects, which can help reduce oxidative stress and inflammation associated with cancer.
- **How to use**: Graviola can be consumed as a fresh fruit, in juice form, or as a supplement (capsules or tincture).
- **Dosage**: Dosages vary depending on the form, but 500–1000 mg of Graviola extract daily is commonly recommended.

Holy Basil (Tulsi) (*Ocimum sanctum*)

Holy Basil, also known as **Tulsi**, is an adaptogen that helps the body cope with stress and reduce inflammation. It is also known for its **anticancer** properties, particularly in preventing the growth of tumors and promoting the death of cancer cells. Tulsi contains **eugenol** and **ursolic acid**, compounds that contribute to its anticancer effects by modulating various molecular pathways.

- **How it works**: Tulsi acts as a potent **antioxidant** and **anti-inflammatory** agent, reducing oxidative damage and inflammation in the body. It has shown promise in inhibiting cancer cell proliferation and preventing the spread of tumors.
- **How to use**: Holy Basil can be consumed as a tea, in supplement form, or as a tincture.
- **Dosage**: Typical dosages of Holy Basil extract range from 300–500 mg per day, or 1–2 cups of tea.

Reishi Mushroom (*Ganoderma lucidum*)

Reishi, often referred to as the "**mushroom of immortality**," has been used for centuries in traditional Chinese medicine for its **immune-boosting** and **anti-cancer** properties. It contains **triterpenoids** and **polysaccharides**, which have been shown to stimulate the immune system, inhibit cancer cell growth, and reduce inflammation.

- **How it works**: Reishi enhances the body's immune response, making it better equipped to fight cancer. It can also inhibit tumor growth, block angiogenesis (the formation of new blood vessels that tumors rely on), and help prevent metastasis.
- **How to use**: Reishi is typically consumed as a powdered supplement, tincture, or in capsules.
- **Dosage**: Standard doses of Reishi extract range from 1000–2000 mg per day.

Detox & Cleansing Herbs

Detoxification, the body's natural process of eliminating toxins, is essential for maintaining health, vitality, and overall well-being. Our bodies are constantly exposed to environmental pollutants, processed foods, chemicals, and stress, all of which can accumulate and affect our health over time. While the liver, kidneys, and digestive system work tirelessly to remove waste, there are times when additional support is needed to help these organs function optimally. This is where **detox and cleansing herbs** come into play.

Herbs have long been celebrated for their ability to aid in detoxification by supporting the body's natural cleansing processes. These herbs work in various ways: promoting liver function, improving kidney health, increasing lymphatic flow, stimulating digestion, and enhancing the elimination of waste through the skin and bowels. By incorporating detox and cleansing herbs into your routine, you can help restore balance, enhance energy, improve digestion, and support your body in eliminating harmful toxins.

Milk Thistle (*Silybum marianum*)

Milk Thistle is one of the most well-known herbs for liver detoxification. The active compound in Milk Thistle, **silymarin**, has potent **antioxidant** and **anti-inflammatory** properties, making it incredibly effective at supporting liver function and detoxification. The liver plays a central role in filtering toxins from the bloodstream, and Milk Thistle can help protect liver cells from damage, enhance the organ's detoxifying abilities, and promote the regeneration of liver tissue.

- **How it works**: Silymarin in Milk Thistle protects the liver from oxidative stress, stimulates the production of bile (which aids in digestion and detoxification), and supports the liver's detoxifying enzymes.
- **How to use**: Milk Thistle can be taken in capsule, tablet, or tincture form. It's also available in tea blends.
- **Dosage**: The typical dosage is 200–400 mg of Milk Thistle extract (standardized to 70-80% silymarin) per day.

Dandelion Root (*Taraxacum officinale*)

Dandelion is often regarded as a **natural diuretic** and **liver tonic**. Its root is particularly effective for stimulating liver function and promoting the production of bile, which aids in digestion and detoxification. Dandelion root has been used for centuries in herbal medicine to help cleanse the liver, kidneys, and digestive system. It can also support the body's natural ability to eliminate excess water, making it an excellent herb for detoxification.

- **How it works**: Dandelion root helps increase bile production, which improves digestion and the breakdown of fats, supporting overall detoxification. It also acts as a gentle diuretic, encouraging the elimination of excess water and toxins via the kidneys.
- **How to use**: Dandelion root can be consumed as a tea, in capsules, or as a tincture.
- **Dosage**: For tea, drink 1–2 cups per day. For tincture or capsule forms, typical doses range from 500–1000 mg per day.

Burdock Root (*Arctium lappa*)

Burdock Root is a powerful detox herb that has been used for centuries to purify the blood and support the liver and kidneys. Known for its **diuretic** and **liver-cleansing** properties, Burdock Root helps remove toxins from the bloodstream and promotes healthy skin by encouraging the elimination of waste through the pores.

- **How it works**: Burdock Root purifies the blood by stimulating liver function and increasing the excretion of toxins through urine and sweat. It also supports kidney function and improves skin health, helping to alleviate conditions like acne and eczema, which can be exacerbated by toxin buildup.
- **How to use**: Burdock Root is commonly used as a tea, in tincture form, or as a supplement in capsules.
- **Dosage**: For tea, drink 1–2 cups daily; for tincture or capsules, follow the recommended dosage, typically 500–1000 mg per day.

Cilantro (*Coriandrum sativum*)

Cilantro, often used as a culinary herb, is also a potent detoxifier, especially for **heavy metals** such as mercury and lead. Cilantro contains compounds that help to bind with and **eliminate toxins** from the body, especially from the liver and kidneys. It is often used in **heavy metal detox protocols** and can also help support digestive health.

- **How it works**: Cilantro acts as a **chelating agent**, meaning it helps bind to heavy metals and other toxins in the body and facilitates their removal through urine and feces. Additionally, it promotes digestion and has **anti-inflammatory** properties that support overall detoxification.
- **How to use**: Fresh cilantro can be added to food, or it can be used in detox smoothies. Cilantro is also available as a tincture or in capsule form.
- **Dosage**: Fresh cilantro can be consumed liberally in meals. For supplements, typical dosages range from 300–500 mg of cilantro extract per day.

Ginger (*Zingiber officinale*)

Ginger, a commonly used root in cooking and herbal medicine, is a powerful herb for detoxification. It is especially useful for supporting digestion, stimulating circulation, and reducing inflammation, which helps the body eliminate toxins more effectively. Ginger is also known for its ability to ease nausea, improve gut health, and boost metabolic function.

- **How it works**: Ginger stimulates the production of digestive enzymes and promotes the movement of waste through the intestines, aiding in digestion and toxin elimination. It also has **antioxidant** and **anti-inflammatory** effects, which support overall detoxification and help reduce the burden on the liver and kidneys.
- **How to use**: Ginger can be consumed fresh, in teas, as a spice in food, or as a supplement.
- **Dosage**: For detox purposes, take 1–2 grams of fresh ginger daily or 500–1000 mg of ginger extract in capsule form.

Nettle Leaf (*Urtica dioica*)

Nettle Leaf is a highly nutritious herb known for its ability to cleanse and purify the blood. It is rich in vitamins, minerals, and antioxidants that support the kidneys and liver in eliminating toxins. Nettle also acts as a **diuretic**, promoting the excretion of waste through urine, which helps in cleansing the body.

- **How it works**: Nettle helps flush toxins out of the body through its diuretic properties while also supporting healthy kidney function. It provides essential nutrients to the body, helping to maintain energy levels during the detoxification process.
- **How to use**: Nettle Leaf is commonly consumed as a tea, or it can be taken in capsule, tincture, or powder form.
- **Dosage**: For tea, drink 1–2 cups daily; for tincture or capsules, typical dosages range from 500–1000 mg per day.

Psyllium Husk (*Plantago ovata*)

Psyllium Husk is a natural **fiber supplement** that supports the digestive system by helping to bulk up stool and promote regular bowel movements. Regular elimination of waste is a key component of the body's detoxification process. Psyllium husk works as a gentle yet effective way to cleanse the colon and improve digestive health.

- **How it works**: Psyllium Husk absorbs water in the intestines, helping to soften stool and make elimination easier. It also helps clear out toxins and waste products from the colon, promoting overall digestive and colon health.
- **How to use**: Psyllium Husk is available in powder, capsule, or husk form. It can be mixed with water or added to smoothies.
- **Dosage**: For powder form, mix 1–2 teaspoons in water or juice and drink once or twice daily. For capsules, follow the dosage instructions on the label.

Yellow Dock Root (*Rumex crispus*)

Yellow Dock is another herb traditionally used to support liver and digestive health. It has powerful **laxative** and **blood-purifying** properties, making it a valuable herb for detoxification. Yellow Dock can help promote regular bowel movements, relieve constipation, and eliminate toxins from the digestive tract.

- **How it works**: Yellow Dock works by stimulating bile production, supporting liver function, and improving digestion. It also helps purify the blood and enhance detoxification by promoting regular bowel movements.
- **How to use**: Yellow Dock is typically consumed in capsule, tincture, or tea form.
- **Dosage**: For tincture, take 1–2 teaspoons daily; for capsules, follow the recommended dosage, typically 500–1000 mg per day.

Heart Health & Circulatory System Herbs

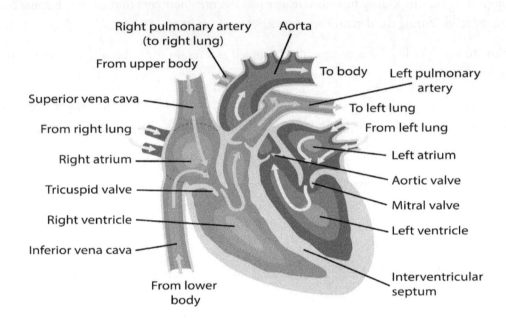

The heart and circulatory system form the vital foundation of overall health, responsible for transporting oxygen, nutrients, and hormones to every cell in the body. Maintaining cardiovascular health is essential not only for preventing heart disease but also for ensuring optimal function of the entire body. Herbs that support heart health and improve circulation have been used for centuries in traditional medicine. Today, many of these time-honored herbs are gaining renewed attention for their ability to enhance heart function, reduce inflammation, lower blood pressure, and improve circulation.

Incorporating heart-healthy herbs into your daily routine can help strengthen your cardiovascular system, reduce the risk of heart disease, and improve your overall well-being. These herbs work in a variety of ways: some reduce oxidative stress, while others support healthy blood vessels, promote blood flow, and help regulate cholesterol levels.

Hawthorn (*Crataegus monogyna*)

Hawthorn is one of the most renowned herbs for heart health. Its use dates back centuries, with traditional medicine recognizing its ability to improve circulation, strengthen the heart, and reduce symptoms of heart disease. Hawthorn is rich in **flavonoids**, **vitamin C**, and **tannins**, which support the cardiovascular system by improving blood flow, enhancing heart muscle function, and lowering blood pressure.

- **How it works**: Hawthorn strengthens the heart muscle, improves blood flow, and dilates blood vessels, making it easier for the heart to pump blood. It has also been shown to reduce **oxidative stress**, which can damage the cardiovascular system, and lower **bad cholesterol (LDL)** levels, further supporting heart health.

- **How to use**: Hawthorn is commonly used in tinctures, capsules, teas, or extracts. It is also available in combination with other herbs for enhanced cardiovascular support.

- **Dosage**: Standard doses range from 250–500 mg of Hawthorn extract, taken 1–2 times daily. For tea, drink 1–2 cups per day.

Garlic (*Allium sativum*)

Garlic is a powerful herb with a long history of use as a natural remedy for heart health. Its active compound, **allicin**, has been shown to lower **blood pressure**, reduce cholesterol levels, and support the cardiovascular system by improving circulation and preventing the formation of blood clots. Garlic's ability to support healthy blood pressure and cholesterol levels has earned it a place in both traditional and modern heart health protocols.

- **How it works**: Allicin and other sulfur-containing compounds in garlic help relax blood vessels, improve blood flow, and reduce blood pressure. Garlic also lowers **LDL cholesterol** and **triglycerides**, while increasing **HDL (good) cholesterol**, thereby improving lipid profiles.

- **How to use**: Fresh garlic can be eaten raw, added to cooking, or consumed as a supplement in capsule or tablet form.

- **Dosage**: For cardiovascular benefits, take 600–1200 mg of garlic extract daily, or consume 1–2 cloves of fresh garlic per day.

Ginger (*Zingiber officinale*)

Ginger is well-known for its digestive benefits, but it also plays a significant role in promoting heart health. Rich in **antioxidants** and **anti-inflammatory** compounds, ginger can help reduce cholesterol, lower blood pressure, and improve circulation. It also acts as a **natural blood thinner**, which can help prevent blood clots and support healthy blood flow.

- **How it works**: Ginger helps reduce **inflammation** and **oxidative stress**, both of which contribute to cardiovascular disease. It also promotes healthy circulation by improving the function of blood vessels and lowering **blood pressure**. Additionally, ginger helps balance **cholesterol levels** by reducing LDL cholesterol and increasing HDL cholesterol.

- **How to use**: Ginger can be consumed fresh, as a spice in meals, or in tea. It is also available in capsule or tincture form for more concentrated doses.

- **Dosage**: For cardiovascular support, take 500–1000 mg of ginger extract daily, or drink 1–2 cups of ginger tea per day.

Cayenne Pepper (*Capsicum annuum*)

Cayenne pepper, the fiery red spice, contains **capsaicin**, the compound responsible for its heat. Capsaicin is not only beneficial for metabolism but also supports cardiovascular health by improving circulation, reducing **blood pressure**, and enhancing the strength of the heart. It has also been shown to improve arterial function and promote healthy cholesterol levels.

- **How it works**: Capsaicin helps stimulate the production of **nitric oxide**, which relaxes blood vessels, improving blood flow and reducing blood pressure. It also promotes fat metabolism and may help lower **LDL cholesterol** while increasing **HDL cholesterol**, contributing to a healthier lipid profile.
- **How to use**: Cayenne pepper can be consumed in food, as a spice, or in supplement form (capsules or tinctures).
- **Dosage**: To support cardiovascular health, 30–120 mg of cayenne extract per day or 1/2–1 teaspoon of cayenne powder in food or tea is recommended.

Turmeric (*Curcuma longa*)

Turmeric is a well-known anti-inflammatory herb, thanks to its active compound **curcumin**. In addition to its potent anti-inflammatory properties, turmeric is highly beneficial for the heart and circulatory system. It helps reduce **oxidative stress**, lower **bad cholesterol** levels, and reduce **inflammation**, all of which contribute to improved cardiovascular health.

- **How it works**: Curcumin in turmeric helps lower levels of **C-reactive protein (CRP)**, a marker of inflammation that is linked to heart disease. It also improves **blood vessel function** and supports healthy circulation by preventing the buildup of plaque in the arteries and improving **endothelial function** (the health of the blood vessel lining).
- **How to use**: Turmeric can be taken as a powder in food, as a supplement, or in the form of a tea. For improved absorption, it is often combined with **black pepper** (which contains **piperine**, a compound that enhances curcumin absorption).
- **Dosage**: A typical dose is 500–2000 mg of turmeric extract daily, divided into 1–3 doses.

Hawthorn Berries (*Crataegus spp.*)

Hawthorn berries are known for their ability to promote heart health and improve circulation. They are rich in **flavonoids** and **anthocyanins**, powerful antioxidants that help protect the heart from damage caused by free radicals. Hawthorn is particularly useful for individuals with cardiovascular conditions, as it strengthens the heart, improves blood flow, and helps manage blood pressure.

- **How it works**: Hawthorn berries help dilate blood vessels, which reduces blood pressure and improves circulation. They also enhance the efficiency of the heart muscle, making it easier for the heart to pump blood throughout the body. Additionally, hawthorn may improve cholesterol levels and reduce the risk of atherosclerosis (plaque buildup in arteries).
- **How to use**: Hawthorn berries are available as a tincture, capsule, or in powdered form. Hawthorn berry tea is also a popular choice.

- **Dosage**: The typical dosage is 250–500 mg of hawthorn extract per day, taken 1–2 times daily.

Ginkgo Biloba (*Ginkgo biloba*)

Ginkgo Biloba is an ancient herb that has long been used to enhance circulation and improve brain function. It supports the circulatory system by increasing blood flow to the brain and extremities, improving oxygenation, and promoting overall vascular health. Ginkgo is also known for its antioxidant and anti-inflammatory properties, which help protect the cardiovascular system.

- **How it works**: Ginkgo improves circulation by dilating blood vessels and reducing blood viscosity. It has been shown to support **endothelial health**, which is crucial for healthy blood flow, and may also help reduce **blood pressure**.
- **How to use**: Ginkgo Biloba is commonly taken as a supplement in capsule or tablet form, or as a liquid extract.
- **Dosage**: Standard dosages typically range from 120–240 mg of standardized Ginkgo extract per day.

Red Clover (*Trifolium pratense*)

Red Clover is often used to support cardiovascular health due to its ability to reduce cholesterol and improve blood circulation. It is rich in **isoflavones**, compounds that have been shown to lower levels of **LDL cholesterol**, improve **arterial health**, and prevent plaque buildup in the arteries.

- **How it works**: Red Clover helps to improve lipid profiles by reducing **LDL cholesterol** and triglycerides while boosting **HDL cholesterol**. It also promotes better circulation and blood flow, contributing to healthier cardiovascular function.
- **How to use**: Red Clover can be consumed as a tea, or it is available in tincture or capsule form.
- **Dosage**: For tea, drink 1–2 cups daily; for tincture or capsules, typical dosages are 500–1000 mg per day.

Fertility and Sexual Health Herbs

Fertility and sexual health are foundational aspects of overall well-being, playing a crucial role in personal health, relationships, and emotional balance. In both men and women, maintaining reproductive health is essential not only for conception but also for overall vitality and quality of life. Today, many people seek natural, holistic approaches to enhance fertility, regulate menstrual cycles, and improve sexual health. Herbal remedies have been used for centuries to support reproductive function and sexual wellness, offering gentle yet effective ways to optimize both.

Herbs for fertility and sexual health work in a variety of ways. Some help balance hormones, regulate menstrual cycles, and improve ovulation, while others support libido, increase sperm count, and promote healthy circulation. These herbs often target the endocrine system, which is responsible for hormone production, and the reproductive system, offering natural solutions to common fertility and sexual health issues.

Red Clover (*Trifolium pratense*)

Red Clover is a powerful herb often used to support both female fertility and sexual health. It is rich in **isoflavones**, plant compounds that mimic the action of estrogen in the body. These compounds help regulate menstrual cycles, improve ovulation, and support hormonal balance. Red Clover is also known for improving circulation, which can support sexual health by enhancing blood flow to the reproductive organs.

- **How it works**: Red Clover helps balance estrogen levels and supports hormonal health, which is key for regular ovulation and fertility. It also enhances circulation, which can increase sexual desire and improve function.
- **How to use**: Red Clover is commonly consumed as a tea, tincture, or in capsule form. It can be used as part of a fertility-enhancing herbal blend.
- **Dosage**: For tea, drink 1–2 cups per day. For tincture or capsules, typical dosages range from 500–1000 mg per day.

Maca Root (*Lepidium meyenii*)

Maca Root, often referred to as "Peruvian ginseng," is a renowned herb for boosting fertility and sexual health, particularly in men. It has a long history of use for improving libido, increasing sperm count, and enhancing overall sexual function. Maca is known for its ability to balance hormones, reduce stress, and enhance energy, which are all factors that contribute to fertility and sexual wellness.

- **How it works**: Maca works as an adaptogen, helping the body adapt to stress, which can often interfere with fertility. It also balances hormones, increasing sexual desire in both men and women and improving reproductive function.
- **How to use**: Maca is typically taken in powdered form (mixed into smoothies or drinks) or as a supplement in capsules or tablets.
- **Dosage**: The typical dosage is 1–3 grams of maca powder per day, or 500–1000 mg of maca extract in capsule form.

Vitex (Chaste Tree Berry) (*Vitex agnus-castus*)

Vitex, also known as Chaste Tree Berry, is one of the most popular herbs for female reproductive health, especially for those struggling with **hormonal imbalances** or **irregular menstrual cycles**. Vitex works by stimulating the pituitary gland, which helps regulate the production of hormones like **progesterone** and **estrogen**, both critical for fertility and reproductive health. It can help women with conditions like **PCOS** (polycystic ovary syndrome), **amenorrhea** (absence of periods), and **luteal phase defects**.

- **How it works**: Vitex helps regulate menstrual cycles, encourages ovulation, and supports the balance of progesterone and estrogen. It is especially useful for women with irregular cycles or luteal phase issues, both of which can impact fertility.

- **How to use**: Vitex is most commonly taken as a capsule or tincture, though it is also available in tea form.
- **Dosage**: For capsules, the typical dose is 400–1000 mg per day. It is important to take Vitex consistently for a few months to see optimal results.

Tribulus Terrestris (*Tribulus terrestris*)

Tribulus Terrestris is a herb that has gained significant attention for its role in boosting sexual health and fertility, particularly in men. It has been traditionally used to enhance libido, improve sperm quality, and increase testosterone levels. Tribulus also supports overall vitality, which can have a positive impact on both sexual function and fertility.

- **How it works**: Tribulus works by increasing the production of **testosterone**, which is essential for male fertility and sexual health. It improves **sperm motility** and **sperm count**, and it also helps regulate sexual desire and performance.
- **How to use**: Tribulus can be consumed in capsule, tablet, or tincture form. It is often included in blends designed to support male reproductive health.
- **Dosage**: A typical dosage ranges from 250–1500 mg of Tribulus extract per day, depending on the form and concentration.

Ashwagandha (*Withania somnifera*)

Ashwagandha, an adaptogenic herb, is a powerful remedy for stress-related fertility issues. Stress can have a detrimental impact on reproductive health, affecting hormone production, ovulation, and sperm count. Ashwagandha helps balance the endocrine system, reduce stress, and increase energy, all of which can enhance fertility and sexual health.

- **How it works**: Ashwagandha works by reducing the levels of cortisol (the stress hormone) in the body. This helps balance overall hormone levels, promoting better fertility and sexual function. It also improves vitality, which contributes to sexual health and well-being.
- **How to use**: Ashwagandha is most commonly taken in capsule or powder form. The powder can be mixed into warm milk or smoothies.
- **Dosage**: The typical dosage of Ashwagandha extract is 500–1000 mg per day.

Dong Quai (*Angelica sinensis*)

Dong Quai, often called "female ginseng," is a traditional herb that has been used for centuries in Chinese medicine to support women's health. It is particularly effective in balancing **estrogen levels**, promoting healthy menstrual cycles, and easing menstrual discomfort. Dong Quai is also helpful in regulating hormones that support **fertility** and in improving circulation to the reproductive organs, which can enhance overall sexual health.

- **How it works**: Dong Quai helps balance estrogen levels, supports the proper functioning of the **reproductive organs**, and enhances blood flow to the uterus and ovaries. It is especially beneficial for women with **irregular periods**, **menstrual cramps**, or **hormonal imbalances**.

- **How to use**: Dong Quai can be taken in capsule, tincture, or tea form.
- **Dosage**: The typical dosage is 500–1000 mg of Dong Quai extract per day, or 1–2 cups of Dong Quai tea daily.

Yohimbe (*Pausinystalia johimbe*)

Yohimbe is a herb commonly used for improving sexual health and function. It is particularly effective for men struggling with **erectile dysfunction** or low libido. Yohimbe works by increasing blood flow to the pelvic region, which can improve sexual arousal and performance. It also has potential benefits for men experiencing low testosterone or sexual fatigue.

- **How it works**: Yohimbe increases blood flow by stimulating the release of **nitric oxide**, which helps dilate blood vessels. This leads to improved blood circulation to the genitals, enhancing sexual performance and arousal.
- **How to use**: Yohimbe is typically available in capsule or extract form. It should be used cautiously due to its potent effects on blood pressure.
- **Dosage**: The typical dosage is 5–10 mg of Yohimbe extract per day, but it is important to consult a healthcare provider before using this herb, especially for those with heart conditions or hypertension.

Saffron (*Crocus sativus*)

Saffron is not only a prized spice in cooking but also a powerful herb for boosting sexual health. It has been shown to improve libido, enhance sexual function, and reduce symptoms of **sexual dysfunction**. Saffron's ability to increase serotonin levels in the brain can enhance mood, reduce stress, and improve overall sexual desire and performance.

- **How it works**: Saffron enhances libido by increasing serotonin levels, which help regulate mood and sexual desire. It also promotes better blood flow to the sexual organs, improving arousal and performance.
- **How to use**: Saffron is commonly available as a supplement in capsule form. It can also be consumed as a spice in food, though its therapeutic dose is generally higher than what is typically used in cooking.
- **Dosage**: A typical dosage for sexual health is 30–100 mg of saffron extract per day.

Antifungal & Antimicrobial Herbs

Infections caused by bacteria, fungi, and other microorganisms are common health concerns that can affect various parts of the body. Whether it's a persistent fungal infection like athlete's foot, or a bacterial infection such as a urinary tract infection (UTI), the need for effective, natural remedies has never been more important. While conventional medicine provides potent antibiotics and antifungals, many people are turning to herbs for their ability to help combat infections naturally, with fewer side effects and a gentler approach.

Antifungal and antimicrobial herbs are known for their ability to fight off pathogenic microorganisms, including bacteria, fungi, viruses, and parasites. These herbs have been used for centuries in traditional medicine systems around the world and have gained increasing recognition for their powerful healing properties. Many of them contain bioactive compounds like **terpenoids**, **alkaloids**, **flavonoids**, and **saponins**, which contribute to their antimicrobial and antifungal actions.

Garlic (*Allium sativum*)

Garlic is one of the most well-known antimicrobial herbs, with a wide range of applications in fighting infections. Its active compound, **allicin**, has been shown to possess powerful antibacterial, antifungal, and antiviral properties. Garlic has been used for centuries in folk medicine for its ability to treat infections and boost the immune system.

- **How it works**: Allicin works by interfering with the metabolism of bacteria and fungi, making it difficult for them to grow and multiply. It also strengthens the immune system, enhancing the body's natural ability to fight off infections.
- **How to use**: Fresh garlic can be eaten raw, added to cooking, or consumed in supplement form (capsules or tablets). Garlic oil can also be used topically for fungal infections.
- **Dosage**: For general antimicrobial support, 1–2 cloves of fresh garlic per day or 600–1200 mg of garlic extract daily is recommended.

Oregano (*Origanum vulgare*)

Oregano, particularly the essential oil derived from it, is a potent antimicrobial herb with well-documented antifungal, antibacterial, and antiviral properties. **Carvacrol** and **thymol**, two key compounds found in oregano, are primarily responsible for its powerful infection-fighting abilities.

- **How it works**: Oregano oil helps to kill harmful microorganisms by disrupting their cell membranes. It has been shown to be effective against a wide range of bacteria, fungi (including Candida), and viruses, including the flu and common cold.
- **How to use**: Oregano can be consumed as a tea, taken in supplement form, or applied topically in diluted essential oil form for fungal infections. Oregano oil is often used as a natural remedy for respiratory infections and digestive issues.
- **Dosage**: For internal use, 100–200 mg of oregano oil extract per day is recommended, or 2–3 drops of diluted oregano essential oil in water or a capsule. Always dilute essential oil before topical use (1-2 drops in a carrier oil).

Tea Tree Oil (*Melaleuca alternifolia*)

Tea tree oil is a powerful antifungal and antimicrobial essential oil that is most commonly used topically. Known for its ability to combat a wide range of pathogens, tea tree oil is especially effective in treating skin infections, such as athlete's foot, ringworm, and nail fungus.

- **How it works:** Tea tree oil contains **terpinen-4-ol**, a compound known to have strong antibacterial, antifungal, and antiviral properties. It works by disrupting the cell walls of bacteria and fungi, preventing them from reproducing and causing infection.

- **How to use:** Tea tree oil is usually applied topically, often diluted in a carrier oil. It can be used to treat skin conditions like acne, fungal infections, and dandruff. It can also be added to bath water or used as a mouthwash for oral infections.

- **Dosage:** For topical use, dilute 2–3 drops of tea tree oil in 1 teaspoon of carrier oil and apply to the affected area 1–2 times daily.

Echinacea (*Echinacea purpurea*)

Echinacea is a well-known herb for supporting the immune system, but it also possesses significant antimicrobial properties. It has been shown to help prevent infections and reduce the severity of cold and flu symptoms. While most commonly used for colds and respiratory infections, Echinacea also supports the body in fighting bacterial and fungal infections.

- **How it works:** Echinacea stimulates the production of white blood cells, which play a key role in fighting off infections. It has both antibacterial and antifungal actions, and it can reduce the severity and duration of infections by enhancing immune function.

- **How to use:** Echinacea is available in tea, tincture, and capsule forms. It can also be taken as an extract to prevent or treat infections.

- **Dosage:** A typical dosage for **preventive** use is 300–500 mg of Echinacea extract daily. For **acute infections**, higher doses of up to 1000 mg per day may be beneficial, but it's important to follow product recommendations and consult a healthcare provider.

Neem (*Azadirachta indica*)

Neem, often referred to as "Indian lilac," is a powerful antimicrobial herb used in Ayurvedic medicine for centuries. It is particularly effective in treating a variety of skin conditions, including fungal infections, acne, and eczema. Neem has antibacterial, antifungal, antiviral, and antiparasitic properties, making it an excellent herb for a range of infections.

- **How it works:** Neem works by disrupting the cell walls of microorganisms, preventing their growth and spread. It is particularly effective against **Candida** infections, **bacterial skin infections**, and fungal conditions.

- **How to use:** Neem is often used in topical applications, such as creams, oils, or in a diluted solution for skin infections. It can also be taken internally in capsule or powdered form for broader antimicrobial support.

- **Dosage:** Neem oil can be applied directly to the skin or diluted with a carrier oil. For internal use, 500–1000 mg of neem capsules per day is common.

Goldenseal (*Hydrastis canadensis*)

Goldenseal is a popular herb with a long history of use for its antimicrobial, antibacterial, and antifungal properties. It contains **berberine**, a powerful compound known for its ability to kill bacteria, fungi, and other pathogens. Goldenseal is often used for respiratory and digestive infections, as well as for skin conditions.

- **How it works**: Berberine in Goldenseal disrupts the cell function of bacteria and fungi, inhibiting their growth. It has been shown to effectively combat a wide variety of infections, including those caused by **E. coli**, **Candida**, and **Staphylococcus**.
- **How to use**: Goldenseal is available as a tincture, capsule, or powder. It can be taken internally for infections or used topically for skin conditions.
- **Dosage**: The typical dosage is 500 mg of Goldenseal extract, taken 1–2 times per day. For **acute infections**, higher doses of up to 1500 mg may be used, but it's important to consult a healthcare provider for guidance.

Clove (*Syzygium aromaticum*)

Clove is a well-known spice that is also a powerful antimicrobial herb. Its active compound, **eugenol**, has potent antifungal, antibacterial, and antiviral properties. Clove is commonly used for toothaches and oral infections but can also be beneficial for fungal infections and digestive issues.

- **How it works**: Eugenol in clove works by disrupting the cell membranes of bacteria and fungi, effectively killing or inhibiting their growth. It also acts as a natural **pain reliever**, which is why it is commonly used in dental care.
- **How to use**: Clove can be used as a spice in cooking, in essential oil form for topical application, or in capsules for systemic infections.
- **Dosage**: For internal use, 500–1000 mg of clove extract or 1–2 drops of clove essential oil (diluted) per day is recommended. For oral infections, a few drops of diluted clove oil can be swished in the mouth.

Lavender (*Lavandula angustifolia*)

Lavender is known for its calming effects, but it also has potent antimicrobial and antifungal properties. Lavender oil is commonly used to treat skin infections, including fungal conditions such as athlete's foot, as well as bacterial infections like acne.

- **How it works**: Lavender essential oil contains **linalool** and **linalyl acetate**, compounds that have antibacterial, antifungal, and antiviral properties. It can help treat infections and promote healing of the skin.
- **How to use**: Lavender essential oil is best used topically, diluted with a carrier oil. It can be used for both fungal and bacterial skin infections and to promote relaxation and healing.
- **Dosage**: For topical use, dilute 2–3 drops of lavender oil in a carrier oil and apply to the affected area.

Liver Support & Detox Herbs

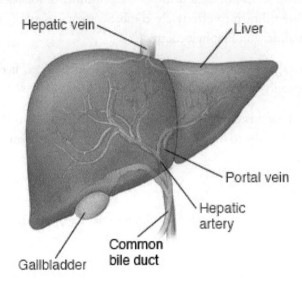

The liver is one of the most important organs in the body, performing a wide range of vital functions, including detoxification, metabolism, and the regulation of hormone levels. It is responsible for filtering toxins from the blood, processing nutrients from food, and storing energy in the form of glycogen. Given the liver's critical role in maintaining overall health, it's no surprise that keeping it functioning optimally is a cornerstone of good health.

However, the modern world exposes the liver to numerous stressors such as pollutants, processed foods, alcohol, medications, and environmental toxins. Over time, these factors can overwhelm the liver, leading to sluggish function, digestive issues, and even liver disease. Fortunately, certain herbs have been used for centuries to support liver health, enhance detoxification, and protect this vital organ from damage.

Liver support and detox herbs help stimulate liver function, promote the breakdown of toxins, and encourage the regeneration of liver cells. These herbs are rich in antioxidants, essential oils, and bioactive compounds that actively protect the liver while promoting its ability to detoxify the body. Incorporating these herbs into your daily routine can help optimize liver function and support your body's natural detoxification processes.

Milk Thistle (*Silybum marianum*)

Milk Thistle is arguably the most well-known herb for liver health, renowned for its ability to support detoxification and liver regeneration. The active compound **silymarin** found in milk thistle has potent antioxidant and anti-inflammatory properties, which help protect liver cells from damage caused by toxins, alcohol, and even certain medications.

- **How it works**: Silymarin helps to stabilize the liver cell membranes, preventing toxins from entering the liver cells. It also stimulates the regeneration of damaged liver tissue and boosts the liver's ability to detoxify harmful substances.
- **How to use**: Milk thistle is commonly consumed as a supplement in capsule or tablet form, but it can also be taken as a tincture or tea.
- **Dosage**: The recommended dosage for milk thistle extract is typically 150–250 mg, taken 2–3 times per day. Standardized extracts (70–80% silymarin) are preferred for optimal results.

Dandelion Root (*Taraxacum officinale*)

Dandelion root, often regarded as a common weed, is a powerful liver-supporting herb. It acts as both a liver detoxifier and a mild diuretic, promoting the elimination of waste through urine and helping the liver process toxins more effectively. Dandelion root also supports bile production, which is essential for fat digestion and detoxification.

- **How it works**: Dandelion root stimulates bile production, which enhances the breakdown of fats and aids in the removal of toxins. It also acts as a gentle detoxifier, promoting the elimination of waste and supporting overall liver function.
- **How to use**: Dandelion root can be consumed as a tea, tincture, or capsule. It is also commonly included in herbal detox blends.
- **Dosage**: For tea, drink 1–2 cups of dandelion root tea daily. For tincture or capsules, the typical dose is 500–1000 mg of dandelion root extract per day.

Turmeric (*Curcuma longa*)

Turmeric is well-known for its anti-inflammatory properties, but it also plays a significant role in liver health. The active compound in turmeric, **curcumin**, is a potent antioxidant that supports liver detoxification by increasing bile production and protecting liver cells from oxidative damage. It is especially beneficial for individuals with chronic liver conditions, such as fatty liver disease or cirrhosis.

- **How it works**: Curcumin supports the liver by stimulating bile flow, reducing inflammation, and protecting liver cells from damage caused by toxins and free radicals. It also helps to break down fats and promotes the healthy regeneration of liver tissue.
- **How to use**: Turmeric can be taken as a powder, in capsules, or as a tincture. Turmeric root can also be used in cooking, such as in curries or smoothies, for a more natural approach.
- **Dosage**: For general liver support, 500–1000 mg of curcumin extract (standardized to 95% curcuminoids) per day is commonly recommended. For the best absorption, turmeric should be consumed with black pepper or healthy fats (such as coconut oil).

Artichoke (*Cynara scolymus*)

Artichoke is not only a nutritious vegetable but also a potent herb for liver detoxification. It has been used for centuries to improve liver health and digestion. The active compounds in artichoke, such as **cynarin**, stimulate bile production and support the detoxification process, making it an excellent herb for those dealing with sluggish liver function or digestive issues.

- **How it works:** Artichoke enhances bile production, which aids in digestion and the elimination of waste products. It also has hepatoprotective properties, helping to prevent liver damage and promote the regeneration of liver cells.

- **How to use:** Artichoke can be consumed as a supplement in capsule form, as a tincture, or as a vegetable in meals.

- **Dosage:** The typical dosage for artichoke extract is 300–600 mg per day, taken in divided doses.

Schisandra (*Schisandra chinensis*)

Schisandra is an adaptogenic herb used in traditional Chinese medicine to support liver health and detoxification. It is often referred to as the "five-flavor fruit" because it has all five basic tastes: sweet, sour, salty, bitter, and pungent. Schisandra is particularly beneficial for protecting the liver from toxic substances and promoting liver regeneration.

- **How it works:** Schisandra contains lignans, which have antioxidant and hepatoprotective effects. These compounds help the liver detoxify harmful substances and regenerate damaged liver cells. Schisandra also improves the body's ability to handle stress, which can further support liver function.

- **How to use:** Schisandra is commonly consumed as a tincture, capsule, or in powdered form. It can also be added to smoothies or teas.

- **Dosage:** The typical dosage of schisandra extract is 500–1000 mg per day. For tea, 1–2 teaspoons of dried schisandra berries can be steeped in hot water.

Burdock Root (*Arctium lappa*)

Burdock root is a traditional herb known for its detoxifying properties. It is particularly beneficial for supporting liver function, purifying the blood, and promoting healthy skin. Burdock root is often included in detox blends to enhance overall liver health and support its natural cleansing abilities.

- **How it works:** Burdock root helps eliminate toxins by promoting the flow of bile and stimulating the liver's detoxification processes. It also has mild diuretic properties, which help the body expel excess waste and toxins.

- **How to use:** Burdock root is available in tincture, capsule, or tea form. It can also be consumed as a vegetable or added to soups and stews.

- **Dosage:** For tea, drink 1–2 cups of burdock root tea daily. For tinctures or capsules, 500–1000 mg per day is typical.

Ginger (*Zingiber officinale*)

Ginger is a well-known herb with a wide range of health benefits, including its ability to support liver detoxification. It has anti-inflammatory and antioxidant properties that can help reduce oxidative stress on the liver and enhance its detoxification capabilities. Ginger also promotes healthy digestion, which further supports liver health by reducing the burden on the organ.

- **How it works**: Ginger stimulates bile production, aids digestion, and reduces inflammation in the liver. Its antioxidants help protect liver cells from damage, while its digestive properties support overall detoxification.
- **How to use**: Ginger can be consumed fresh, in teas, or as a supplement in capsule form. It is commonly used in cooking, such as in teas, smoothies, and curries.
- **Dosage**: For general detoxification and liver support, 500–1000 mg of ginger extract per day is recommended. Fresh ginger root can be added to teas, with 1–2 teaspoons per cup.

Respiratory Support & Cough Remedies

The respiratory system plays a crucial role in our overall health, facilitating the intake of oxygen and the removal of carbon dioxide from the body. However, it is constantly exposed to environmental stressors, allergens, pollutants, and infectious agents that can lead to respiratory issues, such as coughing, congestion, and difficulty breathing. Whether it's the result of a common cold, seasonal allergies, bronchitis, or asthma, respiratory discomfort can have a significant impact on daily life.

Herbal remedies for respiratory support offer a natural approach to easing breathing difficulties, soothing coughs, and improving lung health. Many herbs possess anti-inflammatory, expectorant, antiviral, and antimicrobial properties, which help clear mucus, reduce inflammation, and support overall respiratory function. These herbs can be used to treat both acute and chronic respiratory conditions, as well as to maintain long-term lung health.

Eucalyptus (*Eucalyptus globulus*)

Eucalyptus is widely known for its refreshing, menthol-like scent and its powerful ability to open airways and ease breathing. It contains a compound called **eucalyptol**, which has natural antimicrobial and anti-inflammatory properties, making it an excellent choice for treating respiratory conditions like bronchitis, asthma, and the common cold.

- **How it works**: Eucalyptol works by reducing inflammation in the respiratory tract, loosening mucus, and promoting expectoration (the process of clearing mucus from the airways). It also acts as a natural decongestant, helping to clear nasal passages and ease sinus pressure.
- **How to use**: Eucalyptus oil is commonly used in steam inhalation or added to diffusers for respiratory support. It can also be applied topically (diluted in a carrier oil) to the chest and throat area for relief from congestion.
- **Dosage**: For steam inhalation, add 3–4 drops of eucalyptus essential oil to a bowl of hot water and inhale the steam for 5–10 minutes. For topical use, dilute 2–3 drops of eucalyptus oil in 1 teaspoon of carrier oil and massage onto the chest.

Thyme (*Thymus vulgaris*)

Thyme is an herb with a long history of use in treating respiratory infections, coughs, and bronchial congestion. Thyme's active compounds, including **thymol** and **carvacrol**, give it potent antibacterial, antifungal, and anti-inflammatory properties, making it an ideal remedy for both acute and chronic respiratory conditions.

- **How it works:** Thyme helps to clear mucus from the lungs and soothe irritated airways. It also acts as a natural antimicrobial agent, helping to fight off infections that can cause coughs and other respiratory symptoms.
- **How to use:** Thyme can be consumed as a tea, taken in capsules, or used as an essential oil for steam inhalation. Thyme tea is particularly effective for calming a cough and loosening mucus in the chest.
- **Dosage:** To make thyme tea, steep 1–2 teaspoons of dried thyme in hot water for 5–10 minutes and drink up to 3 times a day. For essential oil use, add 2–3 drops of thyme oil to a bowl of hot water for steam inhalation.

Licorice Root (*Glycyrrhiza glabra*)

Licorice root is a well-known herbal remedy for soothing the throat, reducing inflammation, and alleviating coughs. It has a soothing, demulcent effect on irritated mucous membranes, making it an effective remedy for dry coughs, throat irritation, and respiratory inflammation.

- **How it works:** Licorice root contains compounds that help reduce inflammation in the respiratory tract and thin mucus, making it easier to expel. It also helps to coat and soothe the throat, reducing the urge to cough.
- **How to use:** Licorice root can be taken as a tea, tincture, or in capsule form. It is often combined with other herbs like ginger or slippery elm for added soothing effects.
- **Dosage:** For tea, steep 1–2 teaspoons of dried licorice root in hot water for 5–10 minutes, and drink up to 3 times per day. For tinctures, take 1–2 ml of licorice root tincture (standardized extract) up to 3 times daily.

Note: Licorice should be used with caution, especially for people with high blood pressure or those on certain medications, as it can affect potassium levels and blood pressure.

Mullein (*Verbascum thapsus*)

Mullein is a gentle yet effective herb known for its ability to ease respiratory conditions, particularly those involving congestion and dry coughs. It has anti-inflammatory, soothing, and expectorant properties, making it an ideal herb for clearing mucus and easing irritation in the lungs.

- **How it works:** Mullein acts as a natural expectorant, helping to expel mucus from the lungs. It also soothes irritated airways, reducing coughing and promoting easier breathing.
- **How to use:** Mullein can be consumed as a tea, tincture, or capsule. Mullein leaf tea is especially beneficial for soothing coughs and loosening mucus.

- **Dosage**: To make mullein tea, steep 1–2 teaspoons of dried mullein leaves in hot water for 5–10 minutes and drink up to 3 times per day. For tincture or capsules, follow the recommended dosage on the product label.

Peppermint (*Mentha piperita*)

Peppermint is widely used for its ability to support the respiratory system, especially in cases of nasal congestion, sinusitis, and coughing. The menthol in peppermint provides a cooling sensation that helps to open up the airways, making it easier to breathe and clear mucus.

- **How it works**: Menthol works as a natural decongestant by helping to relax the muscles of the respiratory tract, making it easier to expel mucus. It also has soothing properties that help reduce throat irritation caused by coughing.
- **How to use**: Peppermint can be consumed as a tea, taken as a capsule, or used as an essential oil for steam inhalation. It can also be applied topically to the chest to help open the airways.
- **Dosage**: For tea, drink 1–2 cups of peppermint tea per day. For steam inhalation, add 3–4 drops of peppermint essential oil to hot water and inhale the steam for 5–10 minutes. For capsules, take 200–400 mg of peppermint extract 1–2 times daily.

Elderberry (*Sambucus nigra*)

Elderberry is a powerful immune-boosting herb that is often used to support the respiratory system during colds, flu, and viral infections. It has antiviral properties that help reduce the severity and duration of respiratory infections, and it also supports the body in managing inflammation and congestion.

- **How it works**: Elderberry contains **flavonoids**, which have been shown to help reduce the duration of viral infections, ease congestion, and soothe a sore throat. It also has mild diuretic properties, helping the body flush out toxins and reduce inflammation.
- **How to use**: Elderberry is typically consumed as a syrup, extract, or supplement. It can also be used in teas or tinctures.
- **Dosage**: For elderberry syrup, take 1 tablespoon (15 ml) up to 4 times per day for adults or 1–2 teaspoons for children. For capsules or extract, follow the product's recommended dosage.

Sage (*Salvia officinalis*)

Sage is an herb known for its antimicrobial and anti-inflammatory properties, making it effective in treating respiratory infections, sore throats, and persistent coughs. It has been traditionally used to relieve symptoms of colds, flu, and bronchitis.

- **How it works**: Sage helps to reduce inflammation in the respiratory tract, calm coughing, and fight off bacteria that can cause respiratory infections. It also has astringent properties that help tone the mucous membranes, reducing excess mucus production.
- **How to use**: Sage can be consumed as a tea, used as a gargle for sore throats, or taken as a tincture.

- **Dosage:** To make sage tea, steep 1–2 teaspoons of dried sage leaves in hot water for 5–10 minutes and drink up to 3 times per day. For gargling, prepare a tea and use it as a mouth rinse.

Digestion & Gut Health Herbs

The digestive system is at the core of our overall health. It not only processes the food we eat but also plays a vital role in immune function, mental health, and nutrient absorption. A well-functioning digestive system ensures that we efficiently break down nutrients, absorb vitamins and minerals, and eliminate waste. However, digestive discomforts such as bloating, indigestion, constipation, acid reflux, and irritable bowel syndrome (IBS) are increasingly common due to poor dietary habits, stress, environmental toxins, and other factors.

Herbal remedies offer a natural and holistic approach to improving digestion, soothing discomfort, and supporting overall gut health. Many herbs contain active compounds that can help balance stomach acids, stimulate the production of digestive enzymes, calm inflammation, and support gut flora. These plants have been used for centuries across various cultures to heal digestive issues and optimize gut function.

Ginger (*Zingiber officinale*)

Ginger is a time-honored herb that has been used for centuries to improve digestion, relieve nausea, and ease an upset stomach. The active compounds in ginger, such as **gingerol** and **shogaol**, have powerful anti-inflammatory, carminative, and digestive-enhancing effects.

- **How it works:** Ginger stimulates the production of digestive enzymes, promoting the breakdown of food and improving nutrient absorption. It also has antispasmodic properties that help relax the muscles of the digestive tract, alleviating symptoms of indigestion, nausea, and bloating. Ginger can also aid in the smooth movement of food and gas through the intestines.
- **How to use:** Ginger can be consumed fresh, dried, or in supplement form. Ginger tea is one of the most popular ways to harness its digestive benefits, but it can also be taken as a capsule or in tincture form.
- **Dosage:** For digestive support, drink 1–2 cups of ginger tea daily, or take 500–1000 mg of ginger extract in capsule form 1–2 times per day.

Peppermint (*Mentha piperita*)

Peppermint is widely known for its soothing effects on the digestive system. Its active compound, **menthol**, provides a cooling and relaxing effect on the muscles of the gastrointestinal tract, helping to reduce symptoms of indigestion, bloating, and gas.

- **How it works:** Peppermint works as a carminative, meaning it helps expel gas from the digestive tract and reduces bloating. It also relaxes the muscles of the intestines, helping to ease cramps and discomfort associated with digestive issues. Peppermint can also relieve nausea and help regulate the production of stomach acids.

- **How to use**: Peppermint is commonly used as a tea or in enteric-coated capsules designed to reach the intestines without being broken down in the stomach. It can also be used as an essential oil in aromatherapy or topically for soothing relief.
- **Dosage**: Drink 1–2 cups of peppermint tea per day. If using enteric-coated capsules, follow the dosage instructions, typically 1–2 capsules per day.

Fennel (*Foeniculum vulgare*)

Fennel is a fragrant herb commonly used in traditional medicine to support digestion and alleviate digestive discomfort. Fennel seeds are known for their ability to reduce bloating, gas, and indigestion, making them particularly helpful for those with sluggish digestion.

- **How it works**: Fennel acts as a carminative and antispasmodic, helping to reduce bloating and gas by promoting the expulsion of trapped air in the digestive system. It also relaxes the smooth muscles of the intestines, making it effective for relieving cramps and easing bloating. Fennel can also stimulate the production of bile, improving fat digestion.
- **How to use**: Fennel can be consumed as a tea, taken in capsule form, or used as a spice in cooking. Fennel essential oil is sometimes used for topical massage to alleviate digestive discomfort.
- **Dosage**: To make fennel tea, steep 1–2 teaspoons of crushed fennel seeds in hot water for 5–10 minutes, and drink up to 2–3 cups per day. Fennel capsules typically contain 500–1000 mg of fennel extract, which can be taken 1–2 times daily.

Slippery Elm (*Ulmus rubra*)

Slippery elm is an herbal remedy known for its soothing, mucilaginous properties. It has been used for centuries to treat a variety of gastrointestinal issues, particularly those involving irritation or inflammation of the gut lining, such as gastritis, ulcers, and inflammatory bowel diseases (IBD).

- **How it works**: Slippery elm contains **mucilage**, a gel-like substance that forms a protective layer over the mucous membranes of the digestive tract. This coating helps reduce irritation and inflammation, making it effective for soothing an upset stomach, easing acid reflux, and promoting healing in the digestive system.
- **How to use**: Slippery elm is most commonly consumed in the form of powder or capsules. It can also be taken as a tea or mixed into water to create a soothing slurry.
- **Dosage**: For tea, mix 1–2 teaspoons of slippery elm powder in hot water and sip slowly. For capsules, take 500–1000 mg of slippery elm extract up to 3 times per day.

Chamomile (*Matricaria chamomilla*)

Chamomile is a gentle, soothing herb that has been used for centuries to treat a wide range of digestive ailments. Its anti-inflammatory and antispasmodic properties make it effective for calming indigestion, bloating, and abdominal cramps.

- **How it works**: Chamomile helps to relax the muscles of the gastrointestinal tract, reducing spasms and bloating. It also has mild sedative effects that can help alleviate stress-induced digestive issues. Additionally, chamomile has anti-inflammatory properties that can reduce irritation in the gut.
- **How to use**: Chamomile is most commonly consumed as a tea, but it is also available in capsule or tincture form.
- **Dosage**: Drink 1–2 cups of chamomile tea daily, or take chamomile capsules (typically 300–500 mg) 1–2 times per day for digestive support.

Aloe Vera (*Aloe barbadensis miller*)

Aloe vera is widely recognized for its skin-healing properties, but it also offers significant benefits for digestive health. Aloe vera juice has a soothing effect on the digestive tract and can help ease symptoms of heartburn, acid reflux, constipation, and inflammation.

- **How it works**: Aloe vera contains **acemannan**, a polysaccharide that helps soothe and hydrate the mucous membranes of the digestive tract. This allows it to reduce inflammation, promote healing, and improve overall digestion. Aloe vera also acts as a mild laxative, promoting regular bowel movements.
- **How to use**: Aloe vera can be consumed in juice or gel form. Be sure to choose products that are free from artificial additives and laxative compounds for safer use.
- **Dosage**: For digestive health, drink 1–2 ounces of pure aloe vera juice per day, typically on an empty stomach. Aloe vera capsules can be taken according to the manufacturer's directions.

Artichoke (*Cynara scolymus*)

Artichoke is a powerful digestive herb that helps improve bile production, which is essential for the digestion and absorption of fats. It also contains antioxidants that support liver health, which plays a crucial role in digestion.

- **How it works**: Artichoke increases bile flow, which helps emulsify fats and promote fat digestion. It also has mild diuretic effects, helping the body eliminate excess waste and toxins. Artichoke can support overall digestive function and relieve bloating and indigestion.
- **How to use**: Artichoke is available in capsules, extracts, or as a vegetable in meals. Artichoke tea is also available in many herbal blends.
- **Dosage**: The typical dosage for artichoke extract is 300–600 mg per day, divided into 1–2 doses.

Immunity-Boosting & Immune Support Herbs

A strong and resilient immune system is our body's first line of defense against harmful invaders such as bacteria, viruses, fungi, and toxins. While lifestyle factors such as a balanced diet, regular exercise, and adequate sleep play crucial roles in maintaining immune health, certain herbs have long been recognized for their ability to strengthen immune function, reduce inflammation, and enhance the body's natural defenses.

Herbal remedies have been used for centuries in traditional medicine systems to support and enhance immune activity. These herbs often contain powerful bioactive compounds that help stimulate immune responses, improve circulation, and protect the body from oxidative stress. Whether you're looking to boost immunity during flu season or strengthen your defenses year-round, immune-supporting herbs can be an effective part of your wellness routine.

Echinacea (*Echinacea purpurea*)

Echinacea is perhaps one of the most well-known herbs for immune support, prized for its ability to help prevent and reduce the severity of colds and other respiratory infections. The herb contains compounds called **echinacoside** and **polysaccharides**, which are believed to stimulate the production of white blood cells and enhance the body's ability to fight pathogens.

- **How it works**: Echinacea works by activating various components of the immune system, including macrophages and T-cells, which are responsible for identifying and destroying harmful microorganisms. Echinacea also has anti-inflammatory properties that help reduce inflammation during infections, making it an excellent herb for supporting the body during illness.

- **How to use**: Echinacea can be consumed as a tea, tincture, or in capsule form. It is most effective when taken at the onset of illness or as a preventive measure during peak flu season.

- **Dosage**: To use echinacea as a preventative measure, take 300–500 mg of echinacea extract 2–3 times per day or 1–2 teaspoons of tincture, depending on the product's potency. If using echinacea tea, drink 1–2 cups daily.

Elderberry (*Sambucus nigra*)

Elderberry has gained significant attention in recent years for its potent antiviral properties, particularly in fighting the flu and common cold. Elderberry's active compounds, such as **anthocyanins** and **flavonoids**, help boost immune function by enhancing the production of immune cells and reducing inflammation.

- **How it works**: Elderberry is rich in antioxidants, which help protect the immune system from oxidative stress and cellular damage. Studies suggest that elderberry can reduce the severity and duration of cold and flu symptoms by preventing viruses from entering healthy cells. It also helps to support the body's inflammatory response.

- **How to use**: Elderberry can be consumed in syrup form, as a tea, or in capsules. It is particularly popular as a syrup during cold and flu season.

- **Dosage**: For adults, a common dosage is 1 tablespoon (15 ml) of elderberry syrup, up to 4 times a day during illness, or 1–2 capsules of elderberry extract daily for general immune support.

Astragalus (*Astragalus membranaceus*)

Astragalus is a potent immune-supporting herb with a long history in Traditional Chinese Medicine (TCM). It contains active compounds like **astragalosides**, which help enhance the immune system's ability to recognize and fight infections. Astragalus also has adaptogenic properties, helping the body cope with stress, which can weaken the immune system.

- **How it works**: Astragalus stimulates the production of immune cells such as T-cells and macrophages, increasing the body's resistance to infections. It also has antioxidant properties that protect the immune system from oxidative damage and improve overall vitality. In TCM, astragalus is often used to strengthen the body's defenses and prevent illness, especially during periods of high stress.

- **How to use**: Astragalus is typically taken as a capsule, tincture, or in tea. It is often used as a tonic to strengthen the immune system over time.

- **Dosage**: Take 500–1000 mg of astragalus extract per day, or 1–2 teaspoons of astragalus root in tea. It can be taken long-term for immune support or in higher doses during illness.

Garlic (*Allium sativum*)

Garlic is widely recognized for its ability to fight infections, enhance immune function, and improve overall health. The active compound **allicin**, produced when garlic is chopped or crushed, has antimicrobial, antiviral, and immune-boosting properties that help the body combat harmful pathogens.

- **How it works**: Garlic supports immune health by increasing the activity of immune cells such as macrophages and natural killer (NK) cells, which help fight infections. It also enhances the production of antibodies, which are crucial for recognizing and neutralizing invaders. Additionally, garlic has anti-inflammatory properties that help the immune system respond more efficiently.

- **How to use**: Fresh garlic can be consumed raw, in food, or in supplement form. Garlic capsules or aged garlic extracts are commonly used for immune support.

- **Dosage**: To reap the benefits of garlic, consume 1–2 raw cloves daily, either crushed or chopped. If using supplements, take 600–1200 mg of garlic extract daily. Garlic supplements are available in many forms, including capsules and oils.

Andrographis (*Andrographis paniculata*)

Andrographis is a powerful herb commonly used in traditional Ayurvedic and Chinese medicine to boost immunity and fight infections. The active compound **andrographolide** is known for its antiviral, antibacterial, and anti-inflammatory effects.

- **How it works**: Andrographis supports the immune system by stimulating the production of white blood cells and enhancing the body's response to infections. It also acts as an anti-inflammatory agent, helping to reduce symptoms associated with respiratory infections, such as cough and sore throat.

- **How to use**: Andrographis is typically taken as a supplement in capsule or tablet form. It can also be found in herbal teas or tinctures.

- **Dosage**: A typical dosage is 400–600 mg of andrographis extract daily, taken in divided doses. During illness, the dosage may be increased, but it's important to follow the instructions provided by the manufacturer.

Turmeric (*Curcuma longa*)

Turmeric, with its active compound **curcumin**, is widely known for its potent anti-inflammatory and immune-modulating properties. It supports the immune system by reducing chronic inflammation and promoting a healthy inflammatory response, which is key to fighting off infections.

- **How it works**: Curcumin helps regulate immune cell activity and reduces inflammation throughout the body. By lowering inflammatory markers, turmeric can enhance the body's defense mechanisms and prevent the immune system from becoming overstressed. Turmeric's antioxidant properties also protect immune cells from damage caused by free radicals.

- **How to use**: Turmeric can be consumed as a powder, in supplements, or as a tea. To improve bioavailability, it's best to consume turmeric with black pepper or fat, which enhances the absorption of curcumin.

- **Dosage**: For immune support, take 500–1000 mg of curcumin extract (with black pepper) daily. Alternatively, turmeric tea can be made by mixing 1–2 teaspoons of turmeric powder in warm water or milk.

Reishi Mushroom (*Ganoderma lucidum*)

Reishi mushrooms, known as the "mushroom of immortality," are widely regarded in traditional medicine for their ability to support and balance the immune system. Reishi is considered an **adaptogen**, helping the body respond better to stress while enhancing overall immune function.

- **How it works**: Reishi mushrooms contain **beta-glucans**, polysaccharides that enhance immune cell function, increase the production of antibodies, and stimulate the body's natural defense mechanisms. Reishi is also known for its anti-inflammatory, antiviral, and antioxidant properties.

- **How to use**: Reishi mushrooms are typically taken in extract form or as capsules. Reishi powder can also be added to smoothies or teas for added health benefits.

- **Dosage**: A typical dosage for reishi is 500–1500 mg of extract per day, taken in divided doses. For reishi powder, 1–2 teaspoons per day is a common recommendation.

Brain & Cognitive Function Herbs

In today's fast-paced world, maintaining optimal brain health is more important than ever. Cognitive function—the ability to think clearly, remember important information, stay focused, and make decisions—is crucial for everyday tasks, professional success, and emotional well-being. Unfortunately, factors such as aging, stress, poor diet, lack of sleep, and environmental toxins can impair mental performance and lead to cognitive decline.

Fortunately, nature offers a variety of herbs that have been shown to enhance cognitive function, support brain health, and improve memory, focus, and mental clarity. These herbs work by improving circulation to the brain, reducing inflammation, protecting neurons from oxidative damage, and supporting the brain's ability to form new neural connections.

Ginkgo Biloba (*Ginkgo biloba*)

Ginkgo biloba is one of the most researched and widely used herbs for improving cognitive function. Known for its ability to enhance memory, mental clarity, and overall brain health, ginkgo is often called "nature's brain booster."

- **How it works:** Ginkgo enhances brain circulation by dilating blood vessels and increasing blood flow to the brain. This improved circulation ensures that the brain receives an adequate supply of oxygen and nutrients, which is vital for cognitive function. Additionally, ginkgo contains powerful antioxidants, such as **flavonoids** and **terpenoids**, which protect the brain from oxidative stress and neurodegeneration.

- **How to use:** Ginkgo biloba is commonly available in capsules, tablets, or as a liquid extract. It can also be found in teas, although the concentration may be lower than in standardized supplements.

- **Dosage:** The typical dosage for ginkgo biloba extract is 120–240 mg per day, usually divided into two or three doses. Always opt for a standardized extract (24% ginkgo flavone glycosides and 6% terpene lactones) to ensure efficacy.

Bacopa (*Bacopa monnieri*)

Bacopa, also known as Brahmi, is an adaptogenic herb that has been used for centuries in Ayurvedic medicine to improve memory, learning, and overall brain health. It is particularly renowned for its cognitive-enhancing properties.

- **How it works:** Bacopa works by increasing the levels of **acetylcholine**, a neurotransmitter that plays a key role in memory and learning. It also has antioxidant and anti-inflammatory effects, which protect brain cells from oxidative stress and promote healthy brain function. Bacopa is believed to improve communication between neurons, which enhances memory formation and recall.

- **How to use:** Bacopa is typically consumed in capsule or powder form. Bacopa powder can be added to smoothies or taken with water, while capsules are convenient for regular use.

- **Dosage:** A common dose is 300–450 mg of standardized bacopa extract per day, typically taken in two divided doses. It is recommended to take bacopa for at least 4–6 weeks to experience the full cognitive benefits.

Rhodiola (*Rhodiola rosea*)

Rhodiola is an adaptogenic herb that is known for its ability to combat stress and fatigue, but it also offers powerful benefits for mental clarity and cognitive performance. It is especially beneficial for people facing mental burnout, stress-induced cognitive decline, or the need for improved focus during long periods of mental exertion.

- **How it works**: Rhodiola increases the availability of key neurotransmitters, such as **serotonin**, **dopamine**, and **norepinephrine**, which support mood, focus, and mental energy. It also enhances the body's ability to handle stress by balancing cortisol levels, allowing the brain to maintain its cognitive functions even under pressure.
- **How to use**: Rhodiola is typically taken in capsule or tablet form. It is best consumed in the morning or early afternoon, as it may have stimulating effects.
- **Dosage**: A typical dosage is 200–400 mg of standardized Rhodiola extract per day. It's important to start with a lower dose to assess tolerance, especially if you are sensitive to stimulating herbs.

Lion's Mane Mushroom (*Hericium erinaceus*)

Lion's Mane is a medicinal mushroom that has gained widespread popularity for its remarkable ability to support brain health and cognitive function. This herb is particularly notable for its ability to stimulate nerve growth factor (NGF), a protein that plays a key role in the growth, maintenance, and survival of neurons.

- **How it works**: Lion's Mane promotes neurogenesis, the process by which the brain produces new neurons, and enhances synaptic plasticity, the ability of the brain to adapt and form new connections. This makes it an excellent herb for improving memory, focus, and overall cognitive function, while also offering potential neuroprotective benefits.
- **How to use**: Lion's Mane is available in capsule, powder, or tincture form. It can also be incorporated into food, such as soups or smoothies.
- **Dosage**: A typical dosage is 500–1000 mg of lion's mane extract per day. For the powdered form, 1–2 teaspoons per day is a common recommendation. It's best taken with meals.

Gotu Kola (*Centella Asiatica*)

Gotu Kola is an herb widely used in traditional medicine to promote brain health, improve memory, and reduce mental fatigue. It is considered one of the most important herbs in Ayurvedic and Chinese medicine for enhancing cognitive function and supporting the nervous system.

- **How it works**: Gotu Kola is believed to improve blood circulation, particularly to the brain, which helps enhance cognitive performance. It also helps regulate the levels of **serotonin** and **dopamine**, neurotransmitters essential for mood and mental clarity. Gotu Kola has antioxidant and anti-inflammatory properties that protect the brain from age-related cognitive decline.
- **How to use**: Gotu Kola can be taken in capsule, tablet, or tea form. The herb is also sometimes used in topical preparations to improve circulation and promote skin health.
- **Dosage**: For cognitive support, take 500–1000 mg of Gotu Kola extract per day. If consuming as a tea, steep 1–2 teaspoons of dried Gotu Kola leaves in hot water for 5–10 minutes.

Ashwagandha (*Withania somnifera*)

Ashwagandha is an adaptogen that is particularly beneficial for reducing stress and improving mental clarity. As an adaptogen, it helps the body respond to physical and mental stress, balancing the nervous system and promoting a calm, focused mind.

- **How it works:** Ashwagandha works by reducing the effects of stress hormones like **cortisol**, which can interfere with cognitive function and memory. It also has neuroprotective properties that support the brain's ability to adapt to stress and improve mental endurance. Studies suggest that Ashwagandha can enhance cognitive performance, especially in those experiencing mental fatigue or anxiety.

- **How to use:** Ashwagandha is commonly available in capsules, tablets, or powder form. It is often taken before bed for its calming effects, but it can also be used during the day to support overall mental function.

- **Dosage:** A typical dosage is 300–500 mg of standardized ashwagandha extract per day. If using the powder form, start with 1 teaspoon and increase as needed.

Sage (*Salvia officinalis*)

Sage has been used for centuries not only as a culinary herb but also for its cognitive-enhancing properties. It is known to support memory and concentration, making it a useful herb for mental clarity and focus.

- **How it works:** Sage contains compounds that inhibit the breakdown of **acetylcholine**, a neurotransmitter involved in memory and learning. By preserving acetylcholine levels, sage helps improve cognitive performance, particularly in areas of memory and attention. It also has antioxidant properties that protect the brain from oxidative stress.

- **How to use:** Sage can be taken as a tea, tincture, or in capsule form. The tea is particularly popular as it offers both cognitive benefits and a soothing, relaxing effect.

- **Dosage:** For cognitive support, consume 1–2 cups of sage tea per day, or take 300–600 mg of sage extract in capsule form.

Nervous System & Relaxation Herbs

In today's fast-paced world, stress has become a constant companion for many. Whether from work pressures, personal challenges, or the demands of daily life, chronic stress can take a toll on the nervous system, leading to anxiety, irritability, sleep disturbances, and even physical ailments. Fortunately, nature offers an array of herbs that can help soothe the nervous system, reduce stress, and promote relaxation.

Nervous system and relaxation herbs work by calming the mind, reducing tension in the body, and balancing the nervous system. These herbs have been used for centuries in traditional medicine for their ability to support mental well-being, improve sleep quality, and restore emotional equilibrium. By incorporating these herbs into your wellness routine, you can enhance your body's natural ability to relax, manage stress, and maintain emotional balance.

Lavender (*Lavandula angustifolia*)

Lavender is one of the most well-known and versatile herbs for relaxation, celebrated for its soothing and calming effects on both the body and mind. It has long been used to reduce anxiety, promote restful sleep, and ease muscle tension.

- **How it works**: Lavender contains compounds like **linalool** and **linalyl acetate**, which have a calming effect on the nervous system. These compounds help to lower levels of cortisol, the stress hormone, and stimulate the production of **GABA** (gamma-aminobutyric acid), a neurotransmitter that promotes relaxation and reduces anxiety.

- **How to use**: Lavender is commonly used in essential oil form for aromatherapy, where it can be diffused or applied topically. It is also available as tea, tincture, or in capsule form.

- **Dosage**: For anxiety relief, inhale 2–3 drops of lavender essential oil on a handkerchief or in a diffuser. If using lavender tea, drink 1–2 cups per day. For capsules, take 100–200 mg of lavender extract, up to 2–3 times per day.

Chamomile (*Matricaria chamomilla*)

Chamomile is widely known for its gentle yet effective calming properties. It is often used as a natural remedy to help with sleep, anxiety, and digestive distress. Chamomile's mild sedative effects make it an excellent choice for promoting relaxation without causing drowsiness during the day.

- **How it works**: Chamomile contains **apigenin**, a flavonoid that binds to specific receptors in the brain to promote calmness and relaxation. Chamomile also helps reduce muscle tension and stress by acting as a mild muscle relaxant.

- **How to use**: Chamomile is most commonly consumed as a tea, but it is also available in tincture or capsule form. The tea is particularly popular as part of a calming bedtime routine.

- **Dosage**: To relieve anxiety and promote sleep, drink 1–2 cups of chamomile tea before bed. Alternatively, you can take 200–400 mg of chamomile extract in capsule form, up to two times per day.

Ashwagandha (*Withania somnifera*)

Ashwagandha is an adaptogenic herb that has been used for thousands of years in Ayurvedic medicine to support the body's ability to handle stress. It is particularly useful for balancing cortisol levels and improving the body's response to both physical and emotional stressors.

- **How it works**: Ashwagandha helps the body adapt to stress by regulating the production of **cortisol**, the hormone released during times of stress. It also supports the nervous system by balancing the levels of neurotransmitters such as **serotonin** and **dopamine**, which play key roles in mood regulation and mental well-being.

- **How to use:** Ashwagandha is commonly taken in capsule, tablet, or powder form. It can also be added to smoothies or taken with warm milk.
- **Dosage:** A typical dosage for stress relief and relaxation is 300–500 mg of standardized ashwagandha extract per day. If using the powder form, 1 teaspoon mixed with milk or water is a common dose, usually taken in the evening.

Valerian Root (*Valeriana officinalis*)

Valerian root is a powerful herb traditionally used to promote relaxation, reduce anxiety, and improve sleep quality. It is often used by individuals who experience insomnia, anxiety-related sleep disturbances, or nervous tension.

- **How it works:** Valerian root contains **valerenic acid**, which interacts with receptors in the brain to enhance the activity of **GABA**, a neurotransmitter responsible for promoting relaxation and reducing anxiety. By increasing GABA levels, valerian helps to quiet an overactive mind and calm the nervous system.
- **How to use:** Valerian root is commonly taken in capsule, tablet, or tincture form. It is also available as a tea, though the taste may be strong and earthy.
- **Dosage:** For sleep support and anxiety relief, take 300–600 mg of valerian extract 30–60 minutes before bedtime. For tea, steep 1–2 teaspoons of dried valerian root in hot water for 10–15 minutes.

Lemon Balm (*Melissa officinalis*)

Lemon balm is a member of the mint family and is well known for its mild sedative and calming properties. It is often used to reduce anxiety, relieve stress, and promote better sleep.

- **How it works:** Lemon balm contains **rosmarinic acid**, a compound that has been shown to have anxiolytic (anxiety-reducing) effects. It helps to promote a sense of calm by increasing the production of **GABA** and **serotonin**, neurotransmitters that regulate mood and relaxation.
- **How to use:** Lemon balm is commonly consumed as a tea, tincture, or in capsule form. It can also be used in aromatherapy, where its calming scent helps reduce feelings of stress.
- **Dosage:** For anxiety relief and relaxation, drink 1–2 cups of lemon balm tea daily or take 300–600 mg of lemon balm extract in capsule form. In tincture form, 1–2 ml of lemon balm extract can be taken 2–3 times per day.

Passionflower (*Passiflora incarnata*)

Passionflower is a calming herb often used for reducing anxiety, promoting relaxation, and improving sleep quality. It is particularly helpful for those who experience insomnia or anxiety due to an overactive mind.

- **How it works:** Passionflower works by increasing the levels of **GABA** in the brain, which helps reduce anxiety and promote relaxation. It also acts as a mild sedative, helping the body transition into a calm, restful state.

- **How to use**: Passionflower is typically taken in capsule, tincture, or tea form. It is often used in combination with other calming herbs like valerian or chamomile.
- **Dosage**: A common dosage is 200–400 mg of passionflower extract, taken 1–2 times per day for anxiety or 30–60 minutes before bed for sleep. If using passionflower tea, steep 1–2 teaspoons of dried flowers in hot water for 10 minutes.

Holy Basil (Tulsi) (*Ocimum sanctum*)

Holy basil, or **tulsi**, is an adaptogenic herb revered in Ayurvedic medicine for its ability to reduce stress, enhance mental clarity, and balance the nervous system. It supports both emotional and physical well-being by regulating cortisol levels and promoting a sense of calm.

- **How it works**: Holy basil works by regulating the stress response and supporting overall nervous system function. It enhances the body's resilience to stress and helps restore balance to the autonomic nervous system, which controls involuntary body functions like heart rate and breathing.
- **How to use**: Holy basil is available in capsule, tablet, and tea form. It can also be found as a tincture or powder.
- **Dosage**: The typical dosage for holy basil is 300–500 mg of extract per day, or 1–2 cups of tulsi tea daily. For the powder, 1 teaspoon mixed in water or tea is a common dose.

Anti-Obesity & Weight Loss Herbs

In today's world, managing weight is a common concern for many people. Factors like poor diet, sedentary lifestyles, genetics, and hormonal imbalances can make it difficult to maintain a healthy weight. While exercise and a balanced diet remain fundamental to any weight loss journey, certain herbs have gained popularity for their ability to support metabolism, curb cravings, and enhance fat burning.

Anti-obesity and weight loss herbs can provide a natural, complementary approach to weight management. These herbs work by increasing metabolic rate, suppressing appetite, improving digestion, and supporting fat breakdown. Incorporating these herbs into your daily routine can help optimize weight loss efforts, boost energy levels, and promote overall well-being.

Garcinia Cambogia (*Garcinia cambogia*)

Garcinia Cambogia, often touted as a "miracle weight loss herb," is a tropical fruit native to Southeast Asia. Its popularity stems from its active compound, **hydroxycitric acid (HCA)**, which is believed to play a significant role in weight loss.

- **How it works**: HCA inhibits an enzyme called **citrate lyase**, which is involved in the production of fat. By blocking this enzyme, Garcinia Cambogia helps prevent fat storage in the body. Additionally, it is believed to increase serotonin levels in the brain, which can help reduce emotional eating and control appetite.

- **How to use**: Garcinia Cambogia is most commonly taken in capsule or tablet form. It can also be found in some powdered supplements or as an extract.

- **Dosage**: A typical dosage is 500–1000 mg, taken 30–60 minutes before meals, up to three times per day. Look for a product standardized to contain at least 50% HCA for the best results.

Green Tea Extract (*Camellia sinensis*)

Green tea has long been recognized for its numerous health benefits, and its ability to support weight loss is no exception. Green tea contains a potent combination of antioxidants, including **catechins** and **caffeine**, which have been shown to boost metabolism and increase fat burning.

- **How it works**: The primary active compounds in green tea—**epigallocatechin gallate (EGCG)** and caffeine—work together to enhance thermogenesis (the body's ability to generate heat and burn fat). EGCG has been shown to increase fat oxidation, particularly during exercise, while caffeine provides an energy boost that may help increase calorie expenditure.

- **How to use**: Green tea can be consumed as a beverage, but for weight loss benefits, it is often recommended to take it in concentrated extract form.

- **Dosage**: The typical dosage for green tea extract is 250–500 mg per day, standardized to contain 50–80% catechins, particularly EGCG. For green tea, drinking 2–3 cups per day may also provide weight management benefits.

Cinnamon (*Cinnamomum verum*)

Cinnamon is a flavorful spice that not only adds warmth and depth to dishes but also provides several health benefits, including supporting weight management. It is known for its ability to regulate blood sugar levels, reduce cravings, and improve insulin sensitivity.

- **How it works**: Cinnamon helps stabilize blood sugar levels by slowing down the digestion of carbohydrates. This prevents spikes in blood sugar and insulin, which can contribute to fat storage, particularly around the abdomen. Additionally, cinnamon increases metabolism by improving insulin sensitivity, making it easier for the body to burn fat.

- **How to use**: Cinnamon can be added to smoothies, oatmeal, or tea. It is also available in capsule or powder form.

- **Dosage**: A typical dosage is 1–2 teaspoons of cinnamon powder per day, or 500–1000 mg of cinnamon extract. For best results, use **Ceylon cinnamon**, which is considered the highest quality and safest form of the herb.

Dandelion (*Taraxacum officinale*)

Dandelion is commonly regarded as a weed, but it is actually a highly beneficial herb for promoting healthy digestion and weight loss. It has diuretic properties and can help the body eliminate excess water weight, which may lead to temporary weight loss.

- **How it works**: Dandelion acts as a natural diuretic, helping to flush excess water and waste from the body. By reducing water retention, it may make the body appear leaner, and this temporary effect can encourage continued weight loss motivation. Dandelion also promotes healthy digestion by stimulating bile production, which aids in the breakdown of fats.

- **How to use**: Dandelion is available as a tea, capsule, or tincture. The tea is particularly popular for detox and weight loss purposes.
- **Dosage**: To support weight loss, drink 1–2 cups of dandelion tea per day. If using a capsule or tincture, follow the manufacturer's recommended dosage, typically 500–1000 mg of dried dandelion root per day.

Apple Cider Vinegar (*Malus domestica*)

Apple cider vinegar has become a popular home remedy for a variety of health issues, including weight management. It is believed to support weight loss by controlling appetite, stabilizing blood sugar levels, and improving metabolism.

- **How it works**: Apple cider vinegar contains **acetic acid**, which has been shown to help reduce fat storage and suppress appetite. It also stabilizes blood sugar levels by slowing down the digestion of starches, which helps prevent blood sugar spikes and the subsequent insulin surge that can lead to fat accumulation.
- **How to use**: Apple cider vinegar can be consumed by diluting 1–2 tablespoons in a glass of water, taken before meals. It is also available in capsule form for those who prefer not to drink the vinegar.
- **Dosage**: Dilute 1–2 tablespoons of apple cider vinegar in water and drink before meals, 1–2 times per day. If using capsules, follow the recommended dosage on the product label, usually around 500–1000 mg per serving.

Cayenne Pepper (*Capsicum annuum*)

Cayenne pepper, a member of the chili pepper family, is often used to add heat to foods. It contains **capsaicin**, the compound responsible for its spicy flavor, and it plays a role in supporting metabolism and weight loss.

- **How it works**: Capsaicin has thermogenic properties, meaning it helps the body burn more calories by raising the metabolic rate. It also reduces appetite, making it easier to control food intake. Capsaicin is believed to increase fat oxidation and promote fat loss, especially in abdominal fat.
- **How to use**: Cayenne pepper can be added to meals or smoothies for a spicy kick. It is also available in capsule or tincture form for those who prefer not to consume it in food.
- **Dosage**: A typical dosage is 30–120 mg of cayenne pepper extract per day. If using fresh or powdered cayenne pepper, 1/4–1/2 teaspoon per day is a common starting point.

Forskolin (*Coleus forskohlii*)

Forskolin is an herbal extract derived from the root of the **Coleus forskohlii** plant. It is often used in weight loss supplements for its potential ability to support fat burning and lean muscle mass.

- **How it works**: Forskolin works by increasing the levels of **cyclic AMP (cAMP)** in cells, a molecule that activates the body's fat-burning mechanisms. It stimulates the breakdown of fat cells and enhances the fat-burning process, making it easier to lose body fat.

- **How to use**: Forskolin is most commonly available in capsule form. It can also be found in combination with other fat-burning herbs.

- **Dosage**: A typical dosage for forskolin is 100–250 mg of the extract, standardized to contain 10–20% forskolin, taken 1–2 times per day.

Detoxification & Liver Support Herbs

The liver is often referred to as the body's natural detoxifier, playing a central role in filtering toxins, breaking down waste, and processing nutrients. However, with the onslaught of modern environmental pollutants, processed foods, and stress, the liver can sometimes become overburdened and less effective at carrying out these vital functions. Supporting liver health and promoting detoxification are essential for maintaining overall well-being.

Milk Thistle (*Silybum marianum*)

Milk thistle is one of the most widely studied and revered herbs for liver support. The active compound, **silymarin**, is known for its potent antioxidant, anti-inflammatory, and hepatoprotective (liver-protecting) properties. This herb has been shown to improve liver function, promote cell regeneration, and prevent damage caused by toxins, alcohol, and drugs.

- **How it works**: Silymarin protects liver cells by stabilizing cell membranes and reducing oxidative stress. It also stimulates the production of **glutathione**, a powerful antioxidant that plays a key role in detoxification. Milk thistle may also help improve liver enzyme levels, which can indicate better liver health.

- **How to use**: Milk thistle is most commonly taken in capsule, tablet, or tincture form. It can also be found in powdered form for easy incorporation into smoothies or teas.

- **Dosage**: For liver support and detox, take 200–400 mg of silymarin extract per day, divided into 1-2 doses. For tinctures, 1–2 ml, 2-3 times daily, is a typical dosage.

Dandelion Root (*Taraxacum officinale*)

Dandelion, often regarded as a pesky weed, is a powerful herb for both liver support and detoxification. Dandelion root has been traditionally used to enhance liver and kidney function and stimulate bile production, which aids in the digestion and elimination of toxins.

- **How it works**: Dandelion root acts as a gentle diuretic, helping the body eliminate excess fluid and waste through the kidneys. It also promotes the flow of bile, which is crucial for the digestion of fats and the removal of waste products from the liver. The herb is rich in **antioxidants**, which help protect liver cells from damage caused by free radicals.

- **How to use**: Dandelion root can be consumed as a tea, tincture, or in capsule form. The root can also be roasted and used as a coffee substitute.
- **Dosage**: Drink 1–2 cups of dandelion root tea daily, or take 500–1000 mg of dandelion root extract in capsule form, 1–2 times per day. For tinctures, a typical dosage is 1–2 ml, 2-3 times daily.

Turmeric (*Curcuma longa*)

Turmeric is a well-known spice that has gained widespread acclaim for its anti-inflammatory and liver-supporting benefits. The active compound **curcumin** in turmeric has potent antioxidant and anti-inflammatory effects, making it a valuable herb for liver health and detoxification.

- **How it works**: Curcumin helps detoxify the liver by stimulating bile production, which enhances digestion and helps eliminate toxins. It also supports the liver's natural detoxification enzymes and protects the liver from damage caused by oxidative stress and toxic substances. Additionally, curcumin has anti-inflammatory effects that may help reduce liver inflammation and improve overall liver function.
- **How to use**: Turmeric can be consumed as a spice in cooking, in teas, or in supplement form. To enhance absorption, turmeric is often paired with **black pepper**, which contains **piperine**, a compound that increases the bioavailability of curcumin.
- **Dosage**: For liver support and detox, take 500–1000 mg of standardized turmeric extract (containing 95% curcumin) per day. If using fresh turmeric or powder, aim for 1–3 grams per day.

Schisandra (*Schisandra chinensis*)

Schisandra is an adaptogenic herb traditionally used in Chinese medicine for its ability to support liver function and promote overall vitality. Known as the "five-flavor fruit," Schisandra contains a unique combination of antioxidants, vitamins, and minerals that help detoxify and protect the liver.

- **How it works**: Schisandra contains **lignans**, which have powerful antioxidant effects that protect liver cells from oxidative damage. It also enhances liver detoxification enzymes, improves liver cell regeneration, and increases the production of bile, helping to eliminate toxins from the body.
- **How to use**: Schisandra is available in capsule, tincture, or powder form. It can also be brewed into a tea.
- **Dosage**: A typical dosage of Schisandra extract is 500–1000 mg per day. If using powder or dried berries, 1–2 teaspoons per day is a common dose.

Artichoke (*Cynara scolymus*)

Artichoke, often enjoyed as a vegetable, is also a powerful herb for liver health and detoxification. The leaves of the artichoke plant contain compounds that stimulate bile production and improve fat digestion.

- **How it works**: Artichoke promotes the flow of bile from the liver, aiding in the digestion of fats and the elimination of toxins. It is also rich in **antioxidants** that help protect the liver from damage caused by free radicals and oxidative stress. Additionally, artichoke can help lower cholesterol levels, which benefits overall liver health.

- **How to use**: Artichoke can be consumed as a supplement, extract, or tea. It is also available as a culinary ingredient in many Mediterranean dishes.

- **Dosage**: The recommended dosage for artichoke leaf extract is 300–500 mg, taken 1–2 times daily. For artichoke tea, drink 1–2 cups per day.

Burdock Root (*Arctium lappa*)

Burdock root is a traditional detox herb used to purify the blood and support liver function. It is commonly used in herbal medicine to promote overall detoxification, improve digestion, and enhance the body's natural cleansing processes.

- **How it works**: Burdock root works by supporting liver function and increasing the elimination of toxins through the skin, kidneys, and digestive system. It has mild diuretic properties, which help flush out excess fluid and waste, while its antioxidant-rich profile protects the liver from oxidative damage.

- **How to use**: Burdock root can be consumed as a tea, tincture, or in capsule form. It is also sometimes used in culinary dishes, particularly in Asian cuisine.

- **Dosage**: For detox and liver support, take 500–1000 mg of burdock root extract per day, or drink 1–2 cups of burdock root tea daily. For tinctures, a dosage of 1–2 ml, 2–3 times per day, is typical.

Cilantro (*Coriandrum sativum*)

Cilantro, or coriander, is a common herb used in cooking, but it also offers powerful detoxifying properties. It is particularly effective in supporting the removal of heavy metals from the body, a process known as **chelating**.

- **How it works**: Cilantro binds to heavy metals like **mercury** and **lead** and helps facilitate their removal from the body through the urine. This herb also supports liver health by enhancing detoxification processes and reducing oxidative stress.

- **How to use**: Cilantro can be consumed fresh in salads, smoothies, or juices. It is also available as an extract or tincture.

- **Dosage**: For detox, consume 1–2 tablespoons of fresh cilantro daily, or take 1–2 ml of cilantro tincture, 2–3 times per day.

Blood Sugar Regulation & Insulin Support Herbs

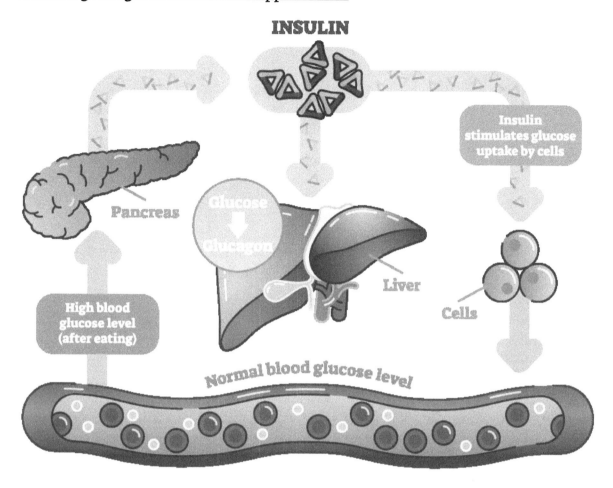

Blood sugar regulation is crucial for overall health, and maintaining balanced glucose levels is particularly important for individuals managing diabetes, prediabetes, or insulin resistance. When blood sugar levels become too high (hyperglycemia) or too low (hypoglycemia), it can lead to a host of complications, including fatigue, dizziness, and in the long term, damage to vital organs.

Cinnamon (*Cinnamomum verum*)

Cinnamon is not only a beloved spice but also one of the most well-researched herbs for supporting healthy blood sugar levels. It contains bioactive compounds such as **cinnamaldehyde** and **polyphenols**, which are known for their ability to enhance insulin sensitivity and regulate glucose metabolism.

- **How it works**: Cinnamon helps increase insulin sensitivity by improving the way the body responds to this key hormone. It may also slow down the digestion of carbohydrates, leading to a more gradual increase in blood sugar after meals. Studies suggest that cinnamon can lower fasting blood sugar levels and reduce hemoglobin A1c (a marker of long-term blood sugar control).

- **How to use**: Cinnamon can be consumed in a variety of ways, including in teas, smoothies, or as a spice in cooking. It is also available in capsule and powder forms.

- **Dosage:** The typical dose is 1–6 grams of ground cinnamon per day, or 500–1000 mg of cinnamon extract, standardized to contain at least 5% cinnamaldehyde. When using ground cinnamon, aim for 1–2 teaspoons per day.

Bitter Melon (*Momordica charantia*)

Bitter melon, a tropical fruit commonly used in Asian and African cuisines, has been used in traditional medicine for its powerful ability to regulate blood sugar levels. Its active compounds, including **charantin** and **momordicin**, have been shown to mimic insulin's effects, helping to lower blood sugar.

- **How it works:** Bitter melon contains compounds that stimulate glucose uptake in cells, increase insulin secretion, and reduce blood sugar production in the liver. It is thought to enhance insulin sensitivity and improve overall glucose metabolism, making it especially useful for individuals with type 2 diabetes or insulin resistance.
- **How to use:** Bitter melon can be consumed fresh, juiced, or in powdered form. It is also available in capsule or tablet form for easier use.
- **Dosage:** For blood sugar regulation, 500–1000 mg of bitter melon extract can be taken 1–2 times daily. If using the whole fruit or juice, aim for 1/2 cup of bitter melon juice or 1 small bitter melon fruit per day.

Gymnema Sylvestre (*Gymnema sylvestre*)

Gymnema sylvestre is a traditional herb native to India and is often referred to as the "sugar destroyer" due to its ability to reduce sugar cravings and support healthy blood sugar levels. It has been used for centuries in Ayurvedic medicine to manage diabetes and improve insulin function.

- **How it works:** Gymnema sylvestre works by reducing the absorption of sugar in the intestines and enhancing the body's ability to use insulin. It is believed to stimulate the pancreas to produce more insulin, while also reducing the sugar receptors on the tongue, which helps curb sugar cravings. Additionally, gymnema may help lower blood sugar levels by increasing insulin sensitivity.
- **How to use:** Gymnema sylvestre is most commonly available in capsule, tablet, or powder form. It can also be found in combination with other herbs for blood sugar support.
- **Dosage:** The recommended dosage is 200–400 mg of gymnema extract, standardized to contain 25–30% gymnemic acids, taken once or twice per day.

Fenugreek (*Trigonella foenum-graecum*)

Fenugreek is a versatile herb that has been used for thousands of years in cooking and traditional medicine, particularly in India and the Mediterranean. It is known for its ability to help regulate blood sugar levels and improve insulin function.

- **How it works:** Fenugreek seeds are rich in soluble fiber, which helps slow the absorption of carbohydrates and reduce blood sugar spikes after meals. Fenugreek also contains compounds like **trigonelline** that enhance insulin secretion and increase glucose uptake in muscle cells. This herb is particularly beneficial for those with insulin resistance and type 2 diabetes.

- **How to use**: Fenugreek can be consumed in the form of seeds, powder, or as a supplement. It is commonly added to soups, stews, and curries, but can also be taken in capsule form.
- **Dosage**: A typical dosage of fenugreek seeds is 1–2 teaspoons per day, or 500–1000 mg of fenugreek extract, taken 1–2 times daily.

Aloe Vera (*Aloe barbadensis miller*)

Aloe vera is widely recognized for its soothing properties, but it also offers significant benefits for blood sugar regulation. Aloe vera gel contains compounds that help reduce blood sugar levels and improve insulin sensitivity.

- **How it works**: Aloe vera works by improving insulin sensitivity and stimulating glucose uptake by cells. Some studies suggest that aloe vera can help lower fasting blood sugar levels and improve blood lipid profiles in individuals with type 2 diabetes. It also helps soothe inflammation, which is often associated with insulin resistance.
- **How to use**: Aloe vera gel can be consumed as a juice or in supplement form. It is essential to use pure aloe vera juice to avoid additives and preservatives.
- **Dosage**: For blood sugar regulation, 1–2 tablespoons of aloe vera juice per day or 500–1000 mg of aloe vera extract can be taken. Aloe vera capsules are also available for easy use.

Turmeric (*Curcuma longa*)

Turmeric, with its active compound **curcumin**, is well-known for its anti-inflammatory properties, but it also offers significant benefits for regulating blood sugar and improving insulin function.

- **How it works**: Curcumin helps reduce inflammation, which is a key factor in insulin resistance. It also increases insulin sensitivity and may help prevent insulin from being inactivated by inflammatory cytokines. In addition, curcumin has antioxidant properties that protect pancreatic cells, which are responsible for producing insulin.
- **How to use**: Turmeric can be consumed as a spice in foods, as part of smoothies, or in tea. For therapeutic use, turmeric is often taken in supplement form for higher bioavailability.
- **Dosage**: The typical dosage is 500–1000 mg of curcumin extract (standardized to 95% curcumin) per day, or 1–3 grams of turmeric powder. To enhance absorption, turmeric is often combined with black pepper extract (piperine).

Holy Basil (*Ocimum sanctum*)

Holy basil, also known as **Tulsi**, is an adaptogenic herb that supports overall health, including regulating blood sugar levels. It has been used for centuries in Ayurvedic medicine for its ability to balance blood sugar and improve the body's response to stress.

- **How it works**: Holy basil helps lower blood sugar levels by improving insulin sensitivity and reducing stress-induced blood sugar spikes. It also has anti-inflammatory and antioxidant properties that help protect the pancreas and other organs from oxidative stress, which can contribute to insulin resistance.

- **How to use**: Holy basil can be consumed as a tea, tincture, or in supplement form. The fresh leaves can also be used in cooking or added to smoothies.

- **Dosage**: A typical dose is 300–600 mg of holy basil extract, standardized to contain at least 2% ursolic acid, taken once or twice per day. For tea, 1–2 cups per day are recommended.

Respiratory Support & Cough Relief Herbs

The respiratory system plays a vital role in our overall health, and maintaining optimal lung function is crucial for our well-being. Whether it's combating seasonal colds, clearing out respiratory congestion, or soothing a persistent cough, herbs have long been used to provide natural support to the respiratory system.

Certain herbs have been studied and valued for their ability to promote healthy lung function, ease breathing difficulties, and alleviate symptoms of coughs, colds, and respiratory infections. These herbs often work by acting as expectorants, soothing irritations, reducing inflammation, and supporting the body's natural immune response.

Eucalyptus (*Eucalyptus globulus*)

Eucalyptus is widely recognized for its powerful ability to support respiratory health, particularly in clearing congestion and soothing coughs. The leaves of the eucalyptus tree contain **eucalyptol** (also known as **cineole**), a compound known for its antimicrobial, anti-inflammatory, and decongestant properties.

- **How it works**: Eucalyptus helps loosen mucus in the airways, making it easier to expel. It also acts as a natural expectorant and decongestant, helping to relieve symptoms of respiratory infections, bronchitis, and the common cold. Additionally, eucalyptus has a cooling effect on the airways, which can help soothe a dry, irritated throat.

- **How to use**: Eucalyptus can be used as a steam inhalation, in topical oils (diluted), or in capsule form. It is also commonly found in lozenges and throat sprays for cough relief.

- **Dosage**: For steam inhalation, add 3-5 drops of eucalyptus essential oil to hot water and inhale the vapors. For capsules, a typical dose is 200-400 mg of eucalyptus extract, taken 1–2 times per day.

Licorice Root (*Glycyrrhiza glabra*)

Licorice root is a time-honored herb used in traditional medicine to soothe respiratory discomfort, ease coughing, and support the immune system. Its soothing, anti-inflammatory, and expectorant properties make it a popular remedy for coughs and respiratory irritations.

- **How it works**: Licorice root acts as a demulcent, coating the throat and respiratory passages to alleviate dryness, irritation, and inflammation. It also supports the immune system and has mild expectorant properties, helping to loosen and expel mucus. Additionally, licorice has mild antiviral and antibacterial effects, which can help support recovery from colds and respiratory infections.

- **How to use**: Licorice root can be consumed as a tea, tincture, or in capsule form. It is often combined with other herbs in cough syrups and lozenges.
- **Dosage**: For licorice root tea, drink 1–2 cups per day. For capsules, a typical dosage is 400–600 mg of licorice extract, 1–2 times daily. If using the tincture, 1-2 ml, 2-3 times daily is common.

Thyme (*Thymus vulgaris*)

Thyme is not only a popular culinary herb, but it also offers significant respiratory support due to its antibacterial, antifungal, and expectorant properties. Thyme has been used for centuries to treat coughs, bronchitis, and other respiratory ailments.

- **How it works**: The active compounds in thyme, including **thymol**, have antimicrobial and soothing effects that help clear respiratory congestion, reduce coughing, and fight off infections. Thyme helps to relax the airways, making it easier to breathe, and also helps loosen mucus, promoting easier expectoration.
- **How to use**: Thyme can be consumed as a tea, tincture, or in capsules. It can also be used as a steam inhalation to help clear the airways.
- **Dosage**: For thyme tea, drink 1–2 cups per day. For capsules, take 200–400 mg of thyme extract, 1–2 times per day. If using tincture form, the typical dose is 1–2 ml, 2–3 times per day.

Mullein (*Verbascum thapsus*)

Mullein is a gentle yet powerful herb for soothing the respiratory system, especially when dealing with persistent coughs, congestion, and irritation. The leaves of the mullein plant contain compounds that help soothe the mucous membranes and support lung health.

- **How it works**: Mullein has natural expectorant properties that help loosen mucus and promote its elimination from the lungs. It also has anti-inflammatory effects, which can help reduce irritation in the respiratory passages. Mullein is especially useful for dry coughs, bronchial irritation, and inflammation caused by asthma or colds.
- **How to use**: Mullein can be consumed as a tea, tincture, or in capsule form. Mullein leaves are also used to make herbal smoking blends that are sometimes used for lung support.
- **Dosage**: For tea, steep 1–2 teaspoons of dried mullein leaves in hot water for 10-15 minutes and drink 1–2 cups per day. For capsules, take 500–1000 mg, 1–2 times per day.

Peppermint (*Mentha piperita*)

Peppermint is widely known for its soothing properties, especially when it comes to digestive health. However, it also offers considerable respiratory benefits, particularly in relieving symptoms of nasal congestion and a sore throat.

- **How it works**: The **menthol** in peppermint provides a cooling sensation that helps clear nasal passages, reduce inflammation, and relieve throat irritation. Peppermint also acts as a mild decongestant and can help relax the muscles in the airways, promoting easier breathing and reducing coughing.

- **How to use:** Peppermint can be consumed as a tea, used as an essential oil in aromatherapy, or taken in capsules.
- **Dosage:** For tea, drink 1-2 cups per day. For essential oils, diffuse 3-4 drops in a vaporizer or add a few drops to a bowl of hot water for steam inhalation. In capsule form, 200-400 mg, 1-2 times per day is typical.

Elderberry (*Sambucus nigra*)

Elderberry has become increasingly popular for its immune-boosting and antiviral properties. It is especially beneficial for alleviating the symptoms of colds, flu, and upper respiratory infections.

- **How it works:** Elderberry contains **anthocyanins**, which are potent antioxidants that support the immune system. These compounds help reduce inflammation in the respiratory tract and enhance the body's ability to fight off infections. Elderberry may also help reduce the severity and duration of cold symptoms, including coughing and congestion.
- **How to use:** Elderberry can be consumed as a syrup, tincture, or in capsule form. Elderberry syrup is especially popular for cough relief during cold and flu season.
- **Dosage:** For elderberry syrup, 1 tablespoon (about 15 ml) of syrup can be taken 1-2 times per day. For capsules, a typical dosage is 500 mg of elderberry extract, 1-2 times daily.

Marshmallow Root (*Althaea officinalis*)

Marshmallow root is known for its soothing, mucilaginous properties, which make it especially useful for calming irritated respiratory tissues and easing coughs. It forms a gel-like substance that coats and protects the throat and mucous membranes.

- **How it works:** The mucilage in marshmallow root acts as a protective barrier, soothing the throat, easing inflammation, and reducing cough reflex. It helps to keep the respiratory tract moist, which is particularly beneficial for dry or persistent coughs caused by viral infections or environmental irritants.
- **How to use:** Marshmallow root can be consumed as a tea, tincture, or in capsule form. It is often combined with other herbs like licorice or thyme for enhanced respiratory support.
- **Dosage:** For marshmallow root tea, drink 1-2 cups per day. For tinctures, take 1-2 ml, 2-3 times daily. For capsules, the typical dose is 500-1000 mg, 1-2 times per day.

Skin Health & Anti-Aging Herbs

Healthy, radiant skin is often seen as a reflection of overall well-being, and taking care of your skin is more than just a cosmetic concern—it's essential for your health. As we age, the skin undergoes changes that can lead to fine lines, wrinkles, dryness, and loss of elasticity. Environmental stressors such as pollution, UV exposure, and poor diet can further accelerate the aging process, causing oxidative damage to skin cells.

Fortunately, nature offers a wide array of herbs that can nourish the skin, protect it from aging, and promote a youthful appearance. These skin-loving herbs provide essential vitamins, minerals, antioxidants, and compounds that support the skin's structure and function. Whether you're aiming to reduce wrinkles, prevent skin damage, or maintain a healthy glow, there are several herbs that can help you achieve your skin health goals naturally.

Aloe Vera (*Aloe barbadensis miller*)

Aloe vera is renowned for its soothing and healing properties, making it a staple in both skincare products and traditional remedies. Rich in vitamins, enzymes, and amino acids, aloe vera is incredibly beneficial for maintaining healthy skin and preventing signs of aging.

- **How it works**: Aloe vera contains **polysaccharides**, which help to hydrate and retain moisture in the skin. It also has antioxidant properties, thanks to compounds like **vitamin C** and **beta-carotene**, which protect the skin from environmental damage. Aloe vera promotes collagen production, helping to maintain skin elasticity and reduce the appearance of fine lines and wrinkles.
- **How to use**: Aloe vera gel can be applied directly to the skin for its soothing and hydrating effects. It can also be consumed as aloe vera juice to support skin health from the inside out.
- **Dosage**: For topical use, apply aloe vera gel directly to the skin as needed. For internal use, drink 1–2 ounces of aloe vera juice daily.

Turmeric (*Curcuma longa*)

Turmeric, with its active compound **curcumin**, is well-known for its anti-inflammatory and antioxidant properties, which can work wonders for skin health. Curcumin helps protect the skin from oxidative stress and supports collagen production, making it a powerful herb for preventing premature aging.

- **How it works**: Curcumin fights inflammation and free radical damage, two of the primary contributors to skin aging. It can help reduce redness, puffiness, and pigmentation. Additionally, turmeric's antibacterial and antifungal properties make it beneficial for acne-prone skin, as it helps to balance oil production and fight breakouts.
- **How to use**: Turmeric can be used in skincare masks, combined with other ingredients like honey or yogurt, to promote skin healing and radiance. It can also be taken internally in supplement form or added to teas and smoothies.
- **Dosage**: For skin masks, mix 1 teaspoon of turmeric powder with honey or yogurt and apply to the face for 10–15 minutes. For internal use, take 500–1000 mg of turmeric extract (standardized to 95% curcumin) per day or drink turmeric tea once daily.

Rosehip Oil (*Rosa canina*)

Rosehip oil, extracted from the seeds of wild rose bushes, is rich in essential fatty acids, antioxidants, and vitamins A and C, all of which play key roles in skin regeneration and anti-aging.

- **How it works**: The high levels of **vitamin A** (retinoids) in rosehip oil promote the regeneration of skin cells, helping to reduce the appearance of scars, fine lines, and age spots. The antioxidants in rosehip oil protect the skin from oxidative stress, while its fatty acids help to hydrate and restore the skin's natural barrier, leaving it soft and smooth.
- **How to use**: Rosehip oil is commonly used as a facial oil, either on its own or mixed with other essential oils. It can be massaged gently into the skin or added to moisturizers and serums.
- **Dosage**: Apply 2–3 drops of rosehip oil directly to the face and neck once or twice a day. It is best used after cleansing and before applying your regular moisturizer.

Ginseng (*Panax ginseng*)

Ginseng is a potent herb used for centuries in Traditional Chinese Medicine for its adaptogenic and rejuvenating properties. When it comes to skin health, ginseng offers a variety of benefits for anti-aging and revitalization.

- **How it works**: Ginseng contains **ginsenosides**, compounds that have been shown to stimulate collagen production, which helps to maintain skin elasticity and reduce the appearance of fine lines and wrinkles. Ginseng also improves blood circulation, which promotes a healthy, glowing complexion. Additionally, its antioxidant properties help protect the skin from oxidative damage.
- **How to use**: Ginseng can be taken as an oral supplement or incorporated into topical skincare products like serums and creams.
- **Dosage**: For internal use, take 200–400 mg of ginseng extract daily. For topical use, apply ginseng-infused skincare products as directed.

Green Tea (*Camellia sinensis*)

Green tea is a powerhouse of antioxidants, particularly **catechins**, which are known for their ability to fight free radicals and protect the skin from damage. Green tea also contains anti-inflammatory compounds that help reduce redness, irritation, and puffiness.

- **How it works**: The antioxidants in green tea, especially **EGCG** (epigallocatechin gallate), have potent anti-aging effects. They help neutralize free radicals, reduce fine lines, and protect the skin from UV damage. Green tea also supports collagen synthesis, which keeps the skin firm and resilient.
- **How to use**: Green tea can be consumed as a beverage or applied topically as a toner or mask. Green tea extract is also commonly found in skincare products like moisturizers and sunscreens.
- **Dosage**: Drink 1–3 cups of green tea daily. For topical use, apply green tea-infused products or use chilled green tea as a toner to refresh the skin.

Lavender (*Lavandula angustifolia*)

Lavender is well-known for its calming effects on the mind, but it also offers significant benefits for the skin. Its antimicrobial, anti-inflammatory, and antioxidant properties make it ideal for soothing irritated skin, reducing acne, and preventing signs of aging.

- **How it works**: Lavender helps balance oil production in the skin, making it useful for both dry and oily skin types. Its antioxidants help protect the skin from free radical damage, and its anti-inflammatory properties reduce redness and irritation. Lavender also promotes the healing of scars and skin tissue.
- **How to use**: Lavender can be used topically in essential oil form (diluted with a carrier oil) or in lotions and creams. Lavender tea is also beneficial for internal calming, which can indirectly benefit the skin by reducing stress.
- **Dosage**: For topical use, mix 2–3 drops of lavender essential oil with a carrier oil like jojoba or coconut oil and apply to affected areas once or twice a day. For internal use, drink 1–2 cups of lavender tea per day.

Calendula (*Calendula officinalis*)

Calendula, also known as marigold, has been used for centuries to promote skin healing and maintain a youthful appearance. This herb is rich in flavonoids, carotenoids, and triterpenoids, all of which are potent antioxidants that protect and nourish the skin.

- **How it works**: Calendula promotes the healing of damaged skin by stimulating collagen production and reducing inflammation. It is often used for its ability to soothe irritation, reduce the appearance of scars, and improve skin tone and texture. Calendula also helps to protect the skin from UV damage and accelerates the skin's natural repair process.
- **How to use**: Calendula can be applied topically in the form of oils, creams, or ointments. It is also available in tincture form and can be added to teas for internal skin support.
- **Dosage**: For topical use, apply calendula oil or cream to the skin as needed. For internal use, drink 1–2 cups of calendula tea per day or take 1–2 ml of calendula tincture, 2–3 times per day.

Hair Growth & Scalp Health Herbs

Hair health is an important aspect of overall well-being, yet it is often impacted by various factors such as genetics, stress, diet, and environmental stressors. Whether you're dealing with thinning hair, dryness, dandruff, or an irritated scalp, certain herbs have been long revered for their ability to promote hair growth, strengthen hair follicles, and maintain a healthy scalp. These natural remedies not only help nourish and rejuvenate the scalp but also stimulate circulation, reduce inflammation, and balance oil production.

By incorporating hair-healthy herbs into your routine, you can enhance hair growth, address common scalp issues, and maintain strong, shiny hair. Below, we explore some of the most effective herbs for supporting hair health and stimulating hair growth, along with their benefits, mechanisms of action, and recommended usage.

Nettle (*Urtica dioica*)

Nettle is a powerhouse herb for hair health, known for its ability to strengthen hair follicles and improve circulation to the scalp. This nutrient-dense herb is rich in vitamins A, C, E, K, and several B vitamins, as well as iron, silica, and calcium—nutrients that support healthy hair growth and overall scalp health.

- **How it works:** Nettle helps promote hair growth by improving circulation to the scalp, ensuring that hair follicles receive the oxygen and nutrients they need to thrive. The high silica content in nettle helps strengthen hair strands, while its anti-inflammatory properties soothe scalp irritation, making it beneficial for conditions like dandruff or psoriasis.
- **How to use:** Nettle can be taken as a tea, tincture, or capsule. It can also be used topically as an infusion or in hair masks.
- **Dosage:** For nettle tea, steep 1–2 teaspoons of dried nettle leaves in hot water for 10–15 minutes, and drink 1–2 cups per day. For capsules, 300–500 mg of nettle extract, 1–2 times daily, is typical.

Rosemary (*Rosmarinus officinalis*)

Rosemary is a popular herb for hair care, known for its stimulating and invigorating effects on the scalp. Rich in antioxidants and anti-inflammatory compounds, rosemary supports healthy hair growth and helps prevent hair loss.

- **How it works:** Rosemary increases blood circulation to the scalp, which helps promote hair follicle activity and encourages hair growth. The herb also contains **ursolic acid**, which has been shown to reduce hair thinning by preventing hair follicle damage. Additionally, rosemary has antimicrobial properties that can help balance the scalp's oil production, making it ideal for those with oily or dandruff-prone scalps.
- **How to use:** Rosemary can be applied topically as an essential oil in hair oils, shampoos, or massaged directly into the scalp. It can also be consumed as a tea or in capsule form.
- **Dosage:** For topical use, dilute 2–3 drops of rosemary essential oil in a carrier oil (such as coconut or jojoba oil) and massage it into the scalp 2–3 times a week. For tea, drink 1–2 cups per day. For capsules, take 200–500 mg of rosemary extract daily.

Saw Palmetto (*Serenoa repens*)

Saw palmetto is best known for its ability to support hormonal balance, particularly in relation to male and female pattern hair loss. This herb has been used in traditional medicine to treat hair thinning and improve scalp health.

- **How it works:** Saw palmetto works by inhibiting the enzyme **5-alpha reductase**, which converts testosterone into **dihydrotestosterone** (DHT). DHT is a major contributor to hair follicle miniaturization, leading to thinning hair. By blocking DHT production, saw palmetto may help prevent hair loss and stimulate the growth of thicker, stronger hair.
- **How to use:** Saw palmetto is commonly taken in capsule or extract form for internal use. It can also be found in topical hair products such as shampoos and conditioners.

- **Dosage**: For saw palmetto capsules, 320 mg of standardized extract, taken once daily, is commonly recommended. For topical use, look for shampoos or hair treatments that contain saw palmetto as an ingredient.

Peppermint (*Mentha piperita*)

Peppermint is an invigorating herb that helps to stimulate hair follicles and improve circulation to the scalp. The cooling and refreshing properties of peppermint make it a popular choice in hair care products for promoting a healthy scalp and stimulating hair growth.

- **How it works**: The menthol in peppermint increases blood flow to the scalp, which enhances the delivery of nutrients and oxygen to the hair follicles. This improved circulation may help to promote hair growth and reduce hair thinning. Additionally, peppermint has antimicrobial properties that help keep the scalp clean and free from excess oil or buildup.
- **How to use**: Peppermint oil can be diluted and massaged into the scalp, or it can be used in shampoos or hair masks. It is also available as an essential oil and can be consumed as peppermint tea.
- **Dosage**: For topical use, dilute 2–3 drops of peppermint essential oil in a carrier oil and massage it into the scalp once a week. For internal use, drink 1–2 cups of peppermint tea daily.

Ginseng (*Panax ginseng*)

Ginseng is a potent adaptogenic herb that not only supports overall vitality and energy but also benefits hair growth by stimulating blood circulation to the scalp and strengthening hair follicles.

- **How it works**: Ginseng enhances the delivery of oxygen and nutrients to the scalp, promoting healthier and thicker hair growth. It has been shown to increase **dermal papilla cells** in the hair follicles, which play a crucial role in hair regeneration. Ginseng also helps combat stress, which is a major factor in hair loss.
- **How to use**: Ginseng can be taken as a supplement or applied topically in the form of hair tonics or oils.
- **Dosage**: For ginseng supplements, take 200–400 mg of ginseng extract per day. For topical use, look for shampoos or serums containing ginseng extract.

Horsetail (*Equisetum arvense*)

Horsetail is a mineral-rich herb that has been used for centuries to improve hair health and stimulate hair growth. It is particularly valued for its high silica content, which strengthens hair and enhances its shine.

- **How it works**: Silica, the main mineral in horsetail, is crucial for healthy hair growth as it strengthens the connective tissues in hair follicles, improving hair structure and elasticity. Horsetail also promotes circulation to the scalp, ensuring hair follicles receive adequate nourishment. Its antioxidant properties help protect the hair and scalp from oxidative stress and free radical damage.
- **How to use**: Horsetail can be consumed as a tea, tincture, or capsule. It is also available in topical products like hair masks and oils.

- **Dosage:** For horsetail tea, drink 1–2 cups daily. For capsules, a typical dosage is 500–1000 mg, taken 1–2 times per day.

Burdock Root (*Arctium lappa*)

Burdock root is a time-tested herb for improving scalp health and promoting hair growth. Rich in essential fatty acids, phytosterols, and inulin, burdock helps balance the scalp's oil production, reduce inflammation, and stimulate healthy hair growth.

- **How it works:** Burdock root supports hair health by promoting better circulation to the scalp and enhancing the detoxification of the skin. The antioxidants in burdock root help to protect the scalp from environmental damage, while its anti-inflammatory properties calm irritation and reduce flakiness. Burdock also helps nourish hair follicles, preventing hair thinning and supporting stronger, shinier hair.

- **How to use:** Burdock root can be consumed as a tea, tincture, or in capsules. It is also available in topical formulations such as hair oils and shampoos.

- **Dosage:** For burdock root tea, drink 1–2 cups per day. For capsules, take 500–1000 mg, 1–2 times daily. For topical use, apply burdock-infused oils to the scalp as directed.